# Desire

# Desire

## THE TANTRIC PATH TO AWAKENING

### Daniel Odier

#### TRANSLATED FROM THE FRENCH BY CLARE MARIE FROCK

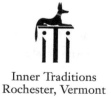

Inner Traditions
Rochester, Vermont

Inner Traditions International
One Park Street
Rochester, Vermont 05767
www.InnerTraditions.com

First U.S. edition published by Inner Traditions in 2001

Originally published in French under the title *Désirs, passions & spiritualité: L'unite de l'être* by Éditions JC Lattès 1999

**Library of Congress Cataloging-in-Publication Data**

Odier, Daniel, 1945-
    [Désirs, passions & spiritualité. English]
    Desire, the tantric path to awakening / Daniel Odier ; translated from the French by Clare Marie Frock.
       p. cm.
  Includes index.
  ISBN 978-0-89281-858-7
    1. Spiritual life—Tantrism. 2. Tantrism. I. Title.

BL1283.855 .O33 2001
294.5'44—dc21

2001016780

Printed and bound in the United States

10

Text design and layout by Crystal H. H. Roberts

This book was typeset in Janson with Bernhard Tango as the display font

The supreme goal of the voyager is to no longer know what he contemplates. Every person, every thing, is an opportunity for a voyage, for contemplation.

**Lao-tzu**

*For Geneviève*

# Contents

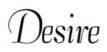

*Desire*

# Part I

*1*

# The Quest: Hedonistic or Spiritual?

$f$or the past few decades, we have been trying in all kinds of ways to liberate ourselves simultaneously from our frenetic materialism and our tired religious traditions. The wave of the sexual revolution affected us; the return in force of the spiritual, in forms most varied, is sweeping over us. The offerings of "personal growth" are multiplying to the point of delirium: Today we have our shaman, our spiritual master, our therapist, our crystal-tarot readers, our clairvoyants, and our Chinese or Tibetan doctors, while in the past we had our family doctor and, for some, our psychoanalyst. The New Age has spawned an array of intertraditional "collages" and has succeeded in turning the authentic mystical movements into the most insipid and illusory of mixtures.

Fortunately, the Tibetans arrived on our shores with their smiles, their sense of humor, their rigor and their profound wisdom—and not only them but also the Sufi masters, the Zen masters, the masters of the different forms of Buddhism, and the Hindu or Amerindian masters who do their best to ensure their marvelous traditions become known in all their authenticity.

The most secretive schools have paved the way up to our present day. The practitioners of *dzogchen*, the Bon-pos, the Naths, the Advaita, and the Aghori are among us. Authentic masters and charlatans daily rub elbows; training programs and retreats are taking place one after another, all over the world. We are learning to walk on fire or to communicate with the spirits, to meditate without moving for twelve hours a day, to go into trances, to breathe like the yogis and yoginis, to do postures, to discover our body and our senses, to have a Tantric orgasm, to recite mantras—unless we fall into the nets of the sects, increasingly hidden yet existing everywhere to channel our dreams of the absolute into a sad alienation from our fundamental freedom. We receive initiations, we have our chakras opened, titillate the kundalini, repeat cabalistic formulas, venerate all the earth deities, converse with the angels, reinvent what little we do know about the traditions into a kind of "ready-to-wear," immediately negotiable package . . . but fundamentally, we are all still looking for the same thing: how to integrate the experience of life in Western society with a deeper consciousness that would bring us bliss and reconcile us with our emotional and sensory natures.

We want a path that would not be opposed to our life; a life that would not be opposed to our path. In short, we want a harmonious integration of the spiritual with the material along an accessible path, one not too estranged from the common culture. We want to attain plenitude without denying life's marvelous effervescence; we want a light and moving joy that would bring us to a larger, more all-encompassing experience of reality.

If we look around, we can see those people who throw themselves into a hedonistic search for pleasure. They try to live out their passions, and sometimes they succeed. They frantically attach themselves to the material world and end up in a state of chronic dissatisfaction, which pushes them to undertake a more and more neurotic quest. These people are often egoistic; they leave a trail of destruction in their wake, yet sometimes we find ourselves secretly envying them because we imagine them to be free. They cause a natural and fundamental longing for pleasure to resonate within us. Their overflowing vitality affects us, even if we feign condemnation of them. Among them, some are touched by grace and discover a more subtle, refined life force in hedonistic enjoyment. Certain of them are deep philosophers.

In opposition to them we find the people who are fascinated by the spiritual search and whose aim is to purify themselves of desires and passions by trying to reduce the impact these have on their daily lives. They are said to be wise or on the path of wisdom. They proudly claim to be of a spiritual school. In observing them we sometimes notice, along with their austerity, signs of coldness and hardness of heart and body; signs of a certain lack of spontaneity. A halo of fear in relation to sexuality encircles their whole being. They seem to have submitted themselves to overly strong tensions; their virtuousness seems a little artificial. Their tolerance has limits, they are often slightly fanatical—indeed, everything about them leads us to believe that their balance is precarious. It would take just one lovely temptation, it seems, to tip them into the neurotic quest for pleasure that they condemn in others. Certain of them succeed in cutting off their passions; they too find a sort of grace and approach what the teachings promised them.

Our cultural and religious heritage seems to tell us that we must choose: the spiritual against the body or the body against the spiritual. D. T. Suzuki, the eminent scholar of Zen Buddhism, one day made this sarcastic comment on the Christian tradition to his friends, American mythologist Joseph

Campbell and psychoanalyst Carl Jung: "Nature against Man, Man against Nature; God against Man, Man against God; God against Nature, Nature against God; very funny religion!"[1]

It is rare that either the hedonistic quest *or* the spiritual quest, with its rejection of the body, brings us happiness, harmony, joy. The language of the mystics almost always aims at reintegrating the vocabulary of passion and love with that of the spirit, which is what makes their language so shocking for puritans. In our Western traditions we have much condemned the impassioned, whether they are people of God or of science, philosophers or artists.

The divorce of our sensory and spiritual natures generates serious problems in adherents of both paths. Traditionally, we assign a period of our lives to try them out, each in turn. With disillusioned smiles, we allow our young people to tempt or try out their passion, desire, and sensorality, knowing that one day they will be like us, weary and well behaved out of obligation.

Certain people doggedly persevere in this search and are thus pitilessly condemned by those who expect everyone to join their ranks. In midlife some people are seized by a brief jolt of passion . . . then they fall back again, exhausted, having become victims of general disapproval. Sometimes this passion revives them and leads them to happiness.

The sexual revolution of the 1960s has been much discussed. It left profound marks on our society, it served the cause of women, and it permitted us to open ourselves to the body, leaving secrecy behind. Today we talk openly about subjects that no magazine would have dared to so much as approach a few decades ago.

In an era where the word *communication* reigns, where an unlimited mass of information can be accessed within a few seconds, we complain about having lost contact with our body and with other human beings. We suffer from extreme solitude, we suffer from no longer touching each other, we suffer from the "virtualization" of our feelings, the expression of our emotions, and our sensorality. AIDS has incited in us such a level of sexual prudence that relationships carry within them the seed of fear and compel us to a superficiality of contact; our bodies scarcely stand a chance of entering into the great expanse of the cosmic play with abandon and creativity.

One day soon this phantom will no doubt be eliminated, and we will know a new period of sexual euphoria, of frenzy, joy, pleasure. Then this cresting wave, too, will turn to calmer waters under the shock of some as yet unknown event, or simply under the weight of its own depletion.

So are we condemned to oscillate unceasingly between these two paths? In just about every person I meet there is a deep intuitive knowledge that a third path does indeed exist. We have suffered too much from fanaticism, violence, and exclusion; we have progressively opened ourselves to the world and its diversity. What men and women seek today is a path that reintegrates these opposites with genuine love and acceptance of all the richness that each human being carries within.

# 2

# A Third Path

From the first centuries of the Common Era, a mystical path whose roots date back at least as far as 3000 B.C.E. revolutionized Hinduism and certain schools of Buddhism. At the time all these traditions were permeated with a fairly acute puritanism and with a striking exclusion of women at the highest levels.

This third path is called Kashmiri Shaivism. Born in the Indus valley five or six thousand years ago, it underwent its most spectacular development in Kashmir and Oddiyana (a neighboring kingdom) and reached its peak between the seventh and thirteenth centuries A.D. Tibetan and Chinese masters of Buddhism and the Indians of the various traditions came to drink from the source in close proximity with the yoginis, women of knowledge who taught the path of the whole person, and with the Siddhas, realized or perfected men and women.

This path, of incomparable depth and subtlety, has nothing to do with the product that the West has commercialized under the name *Tantra*. It is a path whereby a person evolves through sensorality *and* consciousness. It stands in opposition to both the hedonistic sexual quest and the ascetic spiritual quest because it reunites the totality of the person. It is these profound teachings that I propose to introduce to you so that you may discover how to put them into practice in the setting of everyday life—finding joy, ecstasy, and autonomy through being present to reality.

> *Can that be called perfect knowledge . . .*
> *If one is not released while enjoying the pleasures of sense?*[2]

sings Saraha, one of the Buddhist masters who lived sometime between the second and seventh centuries. Saraha became the disciple of a yogini accomplished in the art of shooting arrows into the hearts of people. She belonged to the *sahajiya* school—"awakened adepts of spontaneity." Returning the senses, desires, passions, emotions, and sexuality to the spiritual being is the most profound and the most audacious inner adventure ever imagined by these Buddhist, Hindu, and Kashmiri Tantric masters.

In the beginning the Tantric movement distinctly dissociated itself from the puritan orthodox traditions of Buddhism and Hinduism. It produced such great masters—philosophers, poets, and artists—that Tantric creativity profoundly influenced both the various Great Vehicle Buddhist schools and Hinduism. Numerous historical masters discreetly adhered to the Tantric views. The Vedanta philosopher Shankara, for instance, was a Tantric master. Contemporary Indian figures such as Ramakrishna, Sri Aurobindo, Vivekananda, and Ramana Maharshi—they too were tantrikas. All of Tibetan Buddhism is profoundly Tantric; Chinese Ch'an is permeated with this thinking to such a degree that a female contemporary, master Yuan-tchao, declares that "tantric practise was the crowning of Ch'an."[3] *Dzogchen* has equally influenced and been influenced by Kashmiri Shaivism.

Christianity, Judaism, Islam, Small Vehicle Buddhism, and Hinduism all teach us that we must abandon or sublimate desires and passions in order to carry out a spiritual quest. This puritan position has historically been accompanied by the partial or total exclusion of women from the highest level, that of transmission and teaching.

The different Tantric schools, however, completely reject all formalism, dogmatism, puritanism, eviction of women, and existence of castes. They place the spiritual and mystical path in the social context by abolishing all differences between people. I believe that this profound revolution will blossom into unprecedented creativity in the mystical, scientific, and artistic arenas, a creativity in which each person regains her unity in the total acceptance of her nature.

Far from paving a way that extols the egoistic search for pleasure, the masters of these schools encourage us, through a refined yet playful discipline, not to cut off anything that makes us human, so that we may find a profound way to live our desires and passions by taking them to their ultimate point of incandescence. Attachment and suffering disappear when, as Saraha sings:

> *The faculties of sense subside,*
> *And the notion of self is destroyed.*
> *Such is the Body Innate.*[4]

It is this path—with neither negation nor transcendence— that I have been exploring for thirty years, first with my Tibetan master Kalou Rinpoche, then with my Kashmiri Shaiva master the yogini Lalita Devi. I received permission from the latter to transmit to you this direct and spatial path, that of the recognition of the Self *(Pratyabhijñā).*

Reintegrating desire, the senses, and passion with spirituality is the only serious antidote to religious and sectarian madness or to generalized materialism, because nothing terrifies their adherents as much as these words and the incandescence they point to. These people have a holy horror of anything that cannot be controlled, taken over, or subjugated. And today our desire, our passion, is to find absolute freedom, love, and plenitude without being bound hand and foot. We want to leave behind our ancestral guilt and accept the body wholly: It is our only door into infinite reality. Without the body, we would be nothing. With it, we can be everything.

The American ethnologist Gregory Bateson has also ventured into this complex terrain, which today fascinates a good number of scientists. It consists, Bateson writes, of

> explor[ing] whether there is a sane and valid place for religion somewhere between these two nightmares [the material and the supernatural] of nonsense. . . . I regard the conventional views of mind, matter, thought, and materialism, as totally unacceptable. I repudiate contemporary materialism as strongly as I repudiate the fashionable hankering after the supernatural.[5]

# 3

## Nostalgia for Unity

One of the causes of our suffering comes from the presence, in the deepest part of ourselves, of a kind of nostalgia for unity that sometimes surfaces with great force not only during infancy and adolescence but also in adulthood. This powerful feeling of unity with the world is generally interpreted disfavorably. Adults speak of daydreams, of distraction, of merging states more or less suspicious and destined to disappear over time. And unfortunately this is, in general, how it happens.

We all, at times, go through what are acceptably called crises, in the course of which we once again encounter this powerful nostalgia. Anything that submerges us with force, that makes us doubt our well-regulated life, that carries us away, that touches us deeply, that makes us become conscious of our limits can revive this state of unity—or underline its absence in a disturbing manner. During these crises, we will feel vulnerable but extremely alive, and it is this feeling of drinking once again at the tremoring\* source that will push us to perform sometimes beneficial, sometimes neutral, sometimes catastrophic actions.

This feeling, this need for freedom, this "high" is what we call the passions, and even though we know they give life back to us, they generally trigger in us a certain guilt that goes hand in hand with social disapproval, as if to live is to become progressively used to suffocation, to slow death. No one, not even the paragons of virtue, escapes these jolts, these cataclysms, and if they are most often misinterpreted, it is simply because we all know how essentially marvelous it is to be awakened from our torpor by the passions. Those who have lost this state of grace are the first to condemn the victims of these inner earthquakes, and the misunderstanding continues, carried from generation to generation.

Moralists talk about controlling, reducing, destroying desires and passions, while fanatics take action by destroying the impassioned, but no one can go through life without feeling the devouring substance of desire and passion. Why do these jolts cause us so much suffering? Why, after living through them, do we often return to the state of hibernation? Why do we agree to pay the exorbitant price that society demands of the impassioned? Is there not a fundamental error in the way we orient our lives? Why does our ideal not correspond with our deep intuitive knowledge? Why do we accept that wonder and marvel should no longer be fundamental qualities of our lives?

---

\* Translator's note: Originally *frémissante*, from *frémir*—"to tremor, to quiver, to shudder, to shiver, to thrill, to simmer (as in water)." Daniel Odier uses this word to indicate the idea of *spanda*, which has been translated variously as "the divine pulsation" or "vibration" or "vibratory dynamism of the absolute consciousness." Here, *inner/sacred/divine tremor* or *tremoring vibration* (and their various forms) will be used in the absence of a single English word that adequately conveys this sense of *frémir* and *spanda*.

This abandonment of our potential comes from our up-bringing, education, and socialization; from the difficulties of life; from the need to find our place in it. But above all it comes from our universe of thought, from our mythology, from our religions, from our concepts tied to the biblical texts and to our genesis. Original sin, the fall, and redemption are powerful principles of inhibition and guilt. They condition us to our concept of separation.

It has always been true that those who have authority, in all religions, have tried to retain it by making themselves indispensable and by denying people their own free will and their possibility of being saved if they do not recognize their own inability to deal directly with the divine or, better still, to see the divine in themselves. These intercessors have taken the power and they mean to keep it. They follow the meanderings of social evolution, become more flexible, make reforms, change their image—but fundamentally nothing changes, because the heart of the matter is never broached. They are there to deny our unity with the divine and to make this territory their exclusive hunting grounds. After a few thousand years of varied attempts, it would seem that neither punishment nor heavenly reward has succeeded in giving to people the inner freedom and the plenitude they continue to long for.

If we stop delegating power, however, we liberate ourselves from the absurd expectation that we will be liberated by others. This engenders an immediate impression of space, of calm, thanks to which we become able to examine the situation and once again to take the matter of our potential for freedom into our own hands.

I have used this journey through the unity of being or existence to show to what degree not only the great absolute paths of Tibetan Buddhism, Mahamudra, and *dzogchen* but also that of the original Chinese Buddhism, or Ch'an—paths that saw their beginnings in close proximity to the Siddhas of Kashmir and Oddiyana—converged toward this total acceptance of the absolute nature of the human being in the exploration of a third path marked by the influence of Tantra.

Through the most profound texts of the Tantric tradition, through dialogues with those who follow this path, through questioning of those I meet at the Tantra/Chan center, and through the presentation of the exercises and practices of tantrikas of diverse schools, I propose to accompany you on a journey that will perhaps allow you to verify the intuition or hope most of us carry within: that there does exist a path integrating the totality of the human experience, without fear or taboos, with joy, pleasure, love, and plenitude.

# Part II

# 4

# The Power of Woman

$K$ashmiri Shaivism stands in opposition to Indian tradition because it does not recognize castes and disagrees that mystical teachings and intimacy with the sacred texts be reserved for one of these castes, the brahmans. It disagrees as well with all discrimination between men and women, and all social or ethnic discrimination. Indeed, not only do women have access to the teachings, but Kashmiris have also always believed that their capacities are deeper and more direct than men's. The tradition therefore includes a great number of yoginis and women of knowledge who serve the gods through the exercising of their art, the depth of their practice or their life force, all of which permit them to penetrate the most subtle mysteries. Navjivan Rastogi, an eminent specialist in Kashmiri Shaivism, writes in this regard:

> It may not be entirely out of point to connect this tremendous emphasis on the Shakti aspect [in the Krama system of Kashmiri Shaivism] with the spiritual activity undertaken by the women preceptors. The importance

of the role played by the female teachers may be assessed from the fact that this system is said to have originated from the mouth of the Yoginis (lady ascetics).[6]

Yoginis, like all women, enjoy immense respect from Kashmiris; there is not a single text in which their value is minimized. They are often given the role of mothering the cyclical vision of things, a characteristic of Tantrism, as well as that of a teaching linked to an immediately comprehensible reality—one that knows how to avoid the trappings of a superfluous philosophical sophistication while reaching the greatest depth.

It is also said that Tantrism's attachment to reality rather than to the concept of illusion shared by certain Buddhists (from which Ch'an and the Yogacaras must be excluded) and by the Vedantins is due, in part, to women's vision. For yoginis, there is absolutely no philosophy that cannot be understood and presented clearly to all people. No rituals, dogmas, beliefs, or biases isolate their followers from the rest of the world.

The power of woman finds its origin in the legendary tales where it is told that the gods were troubled by the appearance of a giant phallus that set about destroying paradise. This black stone *linga* was devastating forests and palaces, boring through lakes, filing down mountains and hills. The gods launched their armies against him, but no force could bring an end to the situation. Then the powerless gods remembered the Great Goddess whom, out of vanity, they had been ignoring. They went and bowed before her, made amends, and unanimously recognized her supremacy—on the condition that she put an end to the destructive *linga*. So the Great Goddess manifested herself in the sky, took hold of the giant phallus, and slipped him into her, whereupon he experienced such pleasure that his destructive madness was completely pacified.

Since then, it is said in Tantrism that woman represents power and that man incarnates the capacity for wonder, for marvel. A hymn to the goddess of the *Saktisangama Tantra* honors this creative force:

*Woman is the creator of the universe,*
*the universe is her form;*
*woman is the foundation of the world,*
*she is the true form of the body.*
*Whatever form she takes,*
*whether the form of a man or a woman,*
*is the superior form.*
*In woman is the form of all things,*
*of all that lives and moves in the world.*
*There is no jewel rarer than woman,*
*no condition superior to that of woman.*
*There is not, nor has been, nor will be*
*any destiny to equal that of woman;*
*there is no kingdom, no wealth,*
*to be compared with a woman;*
*there is not, nor has been, nor will be*
*any holy place like unto a woman.*
*There is no prayer to equal a woman.*
*There is not, nor has been, nor will be*
*any yoga to compare with a woman,*
*no mystical formula nor asceticism*
*to match a woman.*
*There are not, nor have been, nor will be*
*any riches more valuable than woman.*[7]

# 5

# We Are What We Seek

*K*ashmiri thought is articulated in a series of simple affirmations:

- You are Shiva-Shakti.
- Shiva-Shakti is the Self.
- The universe is the play of your conscience.

From this, it flows naturally that there is no stain, no purification, no divinity outside the Self; no practice, no ritual, and nothing separate from ourselves to attain. Consciousness is totality; totality is consciousness. The whole quest becomes oriented toward the interior in order to allow the emergence of this unfragmented, perfect, and unalterable consciousness, which is recognized in each one of us. Suddenly there is no longer intercessor, distance, or separation. It thus becomes a matter of freeing consciousness from the opacities that lead us to believe we are separate, solitary, unworthy entities.

Even if we are not obsessed by the divine—which ultimately is but an image of our absolute Self—we find through this quest that the unity we long for is already present within us. What follows is a total easing of the body and mind, a harmony, a profound joy that every human being dreams of experiencing, because everyone knows that happiness is not dependent upon the accumulation of powers or possessions. "You are what you seek," the Tantric masters say.

The quest for this simple bliss, free from dogmas and religious beliefs, from submission to a priesthood, and from the hope of being sanctified by others, is the object of each person's search. This is a secular path *par excellence*. We simply want independence, harmony, a continual and deep enjoyment of the world that no fear or anxiety can tarnish.

The objective is simple. It can be shared by all people, be they materialist or be they attracted to it by spirituality, because this longing for happiness is everyone's. Attaining it is difficult because it will be not submitted to the least romanticism. This longing for happiness is founded on the acceptance of our solitude, thanks to which we will realize that we are connected to everything.

Belonging to groups often generates a kind of narcosis that gives us the illusion of sharing something missing from all the members of the group as individuals: completeness. Our main fear—fear of dissolution, of being nothing—keeps us from realizing that when we think we are one particular thing, and therefore isolated, we indeed become only that thing and lose the rest. In accepting that we are nothing, we gain the world. This logical progression is the key to the Tantric vision and to the creative role of desires and passions, which through our sensorality are seen as the fastest steedlike messengers for leading us to the Self. We must, however, agree on the way in which the tantrikas view desires and passions, and how they live them in an absolute manner.

The first question that bears asking is this: Is it possible to lead our whole lives with passion, and thus avoid feeling the earthquakes of passion's emergence into a life that has previously negated it? Many reasonable people would answer that passion inevitably leads to suffering. Indeed, the word *passion* comes from the Latin *passio*, which means "suffering."

This is a warped view that we are subjected to from a very early age. Adding to it is the fact that in general, those who attempt the experience of continual passion get burned, suffer, and fade away. We lack therefore any convincing examples and decide that it is more prudent to enter the passionate spheres only in those brief, inevitable moments when they overwhelm us, at which point we will draw from these life reservoirs in a despairing, hopeless way.

These violently abrupt changes exhaust us. The Tantric vision, on the other hand, is made of continuity in experience.

We have all experienced the profound inner tremoring of existence for a few seconds or a few hours. If we examine our past, we will remember having been, during our childhood or adolescence, completely connected to the world. Remembering this ecstatic communion with a person or an object will prepare us to go farther in accepting the passion of existence.

The more I immerse myself in Tantrism, the more I feel it is possible to find, in our culture as well, traces of this freedom, of this return to the source of existence, to simplicity, to the fundamental experience of the *I Am* that all people can share. There is no doubt for me that this manner of gliding toward freedom and original ecstasy through the senses, desire, and passion can find echoes of itself in all the traditions when they are deeply understood.

If I have chosen to plunge into the Kashmiri tradition, it is simply because this seemed to me the most direct path. To a degree I have also followed it because it was incarnated by a woman, the yogini Lalita Devi. I saw in this tradition a tribute to our most anciently held memory, the divinity of woman, and likewise an homage to today's woman, who carries this divinity within her and is able to transmit the deep feeling of this divinity to the sensitive and wonder-filled men whom she welcomes into her body.

Thus, in presenting the principles of the Kashmiri path in relation to the senses, desires, and passions, my hope is that I might revive this memory in those belonging to other traditions so that they may meet in their own sources this remarkable life force and integrate it into their daily lives with total presence to reality.

# 6

## Breath:
## Door of Our Sensorality

*I*f presence to sensations, emotions, and thoughts is to reach plenitude, everything must start with awareness of the breath. Rather than devoting ourselves from the start to breathing exercises, the Tantric masters advise us to become conscious of the manner in which we breathe. This one act of consciousness will calm and deepen the breath. There are never any new behaviors to apply, because the masters believe that nothing deep can be developed starting from the unconscious.

When we have become conscious of our way of breathing, we can allow the breath to find its proper place and its plenitude, very progressively encouraging complete breathing—on the condition that the process be founded on the emergence of consciousness and not on the idea of "doing," of applying a technique to obtain an effect. Nothing is done in Tantric yoga to obtain some future gratification; on the contrary, it offers "practices" whose fruits are immediately present in "the practice" itself. In this way we breathe solely to experience the profound harmony of breathing—nothing else.

*Every morning, as soon as I awaken, while still in bed, I bring my awareness to my abdominal breathing and my pelvis. Perfectly at ease and relaxed, hands on my chest, fingers on my sternum, legs open, I feel my abdominal muscles relaxing as I gently and peacefully inhale while I fill my belly, releasing the sacrum backward and arching my lower back with the inhalation.*

*After a slight pause, I exhale, drawing my stomach muscles back in and pushing my sacrum forward as if I were making love to a goddess or a god.*

*Gradually, I become conscious of the effects of this breathing on my diaphragm, which undulates like a jellyfish in the warm waters of the ocean.*

*After a few weeks of this awareness of my breath—which develops into conscious breathing—I regularly become conscious of this breathing again and again, and I allow it to blossom and open when I leave my home, when I walk down the street, when I arrive at work, when a natural break occurs between two moments of concentration.*

*Whenever I have to go from one place to another, I use this movement to my benefit by taking a few steps while deeply feeling my breath.*

*When I take a break for lunch, I again put myself in consciousness of my breath.*

*Before an important meeting, I "place myself" through abdominal breathing. During the meeting, I return regularly to my breath, I allow my pelvis to relax, I release my muscles deeply.*

It is much more important to become conscious of the breath many times a day than to attempt to practice for too long at a time. All the "micropractices" of Tantric yoga[8] are done for five, ten, or thirty seconds followed by a conscious return to the habitual manner of living or doing things. This pulling back or withdrawing of attention is crucial, because it allows us not to get lost in automatic activity while believing we are doing our practice.

At first, I try to be present to my breath ten to twenty times a day. Little by little, to the degree that this awareness brings me pleasure, I let the number of times I become aware of the breath increase to a hundred times a day and more. Pleasure is an essential element of Tantric practice, because once we find pleasure in presence, we have a natural tendency to return to it. It is thus no longer a practice but a way in which to savor life and our sensorality more fully, and this is the basis of all the subsequent practices.

The effects of conscious breathing or partially conscious breathing are extraordinary:

- Decrease in stress
- Development of sensory sensitivity
- More regular sleep
- General equilibrium of the body
- Regular blood and lymph flow
- Calmness, equilibrium
- Improved mental capacity
- Mini rests distilled over the whole of the day
- Improved concentration
- More precise physical movements
- Feelings of plenitude and joy

Once conscious breathing replaces automatic breathing, you will feel a complete change in your way of perceiving the world. Fears and anxieties about relationships with others will disappear; you will have a profound feeling of being connected to the earth, the impression that we call "having your feet on the ground."

The success of the later practices, all of which deal with full consciousness of the sensations, depends uniquely upon the ability to breathe consciously. This is so important that certain Tantric masters limit their teachings to the practice of breathing. The Buddha himself, in the *Anapanasati Sutra*, bases his teaching on the practice of full consciousness of the breath: "The practice of Full Awareness of Breathing, if developed and practiced continuously, will lead to perfect accomplishment. . . ."[9] The great seventeenth-century Zen master Man-An wrote, in his "Elementary Talk on Zen":

> When you breathe out, know you are breathing out; when you breathe in, know you are breathing in. Focus your consciousness on your breathing, not letting consciousness go up or down or out or in, not thinking discursively, not making intellectual or emotional interpretations, not trying to figure anything out, simply being aware of outgoing and incoming breath, not missing a single breath.[10]

# 7

# Experiencing Totality: First Experience?

Where does it come from, this intuition we have that there could be identity between us and the world? No one suggested it to us; no one has supported us when we have expressed our feelings or intuitions about unity. Why do we persist so determinedly in thinking that this union is possible? Quite simply, it is because we have had a direct, intimate experience of it and so our certainty is inalienable. We lived this experience well before our conditioning took place.

During the first weeks of his life, the newborn does not feel separate from his mother or his surroundings; he is in undifferentiated unity. These are probably the most troubling and the most powerful moments of our lives. No other feeling will ever replace the primary importance of this experience. It is as if this experience is engraved in us, whatever paths we follow. Sometimes, this feeling will resurge unexpectedly and remind us for our whole life that we can again communicate with it.

Freud called this the oceanic feeling. "One may . . . rightly call oneself religious on the ground of this oceanic feeling alone," he added, "even if one rejects every belief and every illusion."[11]

This sensation of unity against which we will struggle seems to be our first experience as human beings. If we could go back in time, we would doubtless perceive that this sensation has always been the foundation of the human experience, for as far back as we can go, and that it is still inscribed in our brain, in our genes.

Today we know that the brain, before birth, has as many neurons as there are constellations in space—approximately one hundred billion, each of which can establish twenty thousand connections. Very quickly, these neurons begin a process of destruction that will allow the brain to function; over the course of a lifetime, 90 percent of them will be destroyed.*
It is a little as if our brain contained the totality of the universe and loses this totality in the interest of being able to function—but the traces that remain leave in us a nostalgia for the whole.

But the development of this idea of separation, more cultural than personal, is it inevitable? While the ego develops—very early on, well before the appearance of language—there appears along with it the feeling of separateness, which the tone of our whole culture will accelerate. We must distinguish ourselves, we must rise to challenges, show how brilliant and competent we are—and none of this happens without inflation of the ego. How does it happen, then, that when we have fulfilled all these functions with brio, this nostalgia for unity still affects us? It is simply because this is our essential nature; we can no more forget it than we can forget to breathe. It is upon this central observation that the whole flexible and spherical structure of Kashmiri Shaivism is built.

---

* Even after 90 percent of our neurons are destroyed, however, it is worth noting that enough remain to establish two million billion neural connections.

# 8

*Touching the World*

The skin demarks the visible limit of the body and the point of contact with the world. Through the breath, you will realize that your skin has become more alive, quivering, softer. After a few weeks of presence to your breath, you will discover that your body is not limited by the skin. Your sensations will extend well beyond the skin, in a succession of waves that will seem to go fairly far from you, touch the world, and then return close to your body. This sensation is extremely pleasant and is what all yoginis and yogis feel.

The skin represents around 16 percent of the weight of our body and covers more than one and a half square meters. It is our most sensitive organ, the one that "nourishes" us most. The health of a newborn who is not touched, even if fed, will rapidly decline; she will develop cerebral problems and can even die. Adults who do not touch and are not touched become pale and sickly, drained of life. Sometimes physical contact gives life back to the ill; certain nurses know this well. Massages are one of the most efficient ways to stay in good health and to maintain a well-balanced nervous system in the continual rediscovery of our body. African and Asian women massage their babies a lot to get all the branches of their nervous systems working. They readily tell us, to use a common expression, that they "finish" their babies, because they deeply feel that the process of entering the world is not completed with the physical birth. Today we know that brain circuits that are not stimulated during the first few months of life automatically self-destruct.

A simple caress starts our whole sensory system working. Tantrikas practice massage their whole lives because, for them, the Kashmiri art of touching is considered a wholly unique yoga unto itself. It is the gateway to our sensorality and stimulates a person to constant creativity.

The Kashmiri masters speak of the preeminence of the sense of touch. For them, a human being naturally recovers his unity when he is touched deeply—that is, when contact is no longer a sexual strategy. When nothing is "wanted." This kind of contact is established within a sort of grace, because it gives back to anyone touched in this way a sense of his own spatiality. The master's touch is spoken of in numerous poems: It restores this marvelous sensation of receiving a selfless gesture, stripped of all projection.

To touch another in this way necessitates simply being the other, and to be the other necessitates living in a state of nonduality. To have been touched in this way restores to the body its sacred vibration and will sometimes render it intolerably sensitive to all the "programmed" contact of unaware partners. From that moment on, the body will insist on being approached with veneration and true presence.

*As soon as I wake up, I become conscious of my skin—the soft, thin membrane that marks the limits of me. What sensations does my skin feel? Warmth, well-being, ease?*

*I get up; the temperature changes. How does my skin react? I cross a room, I feel the contact of my feet on the floor, my hand touches a doorknob, I open the door, I am alive.*

*I have prepared my breakfast. I touch things with different textures, different temperatures. Bread, knife, full cup, and so forth.*

*I take a shower. The whole of my skin is now touched by the streams of hot water. If I am absent, unaware, the satisfaction is mediocre; it is an obligatory passage from one act to the next. If I am present, my whole body will find life, the deep satisfaction of feeling these wonderful sensations of water drops projected onto my skin.*

*The whole day, my skin will change environments, respond to all kinds of stimulation. This life of continuous tremoring is the life of the yoga of awareness and consciousness. To open myself to this life is to practice. To accept that I am a wholly exceptional and unique living being. To emerge from the automatism that brings me absolutely no satisfaction.*

To learn to enjoy simple pleasures is to decondition ourselves gradually from our quest for intense pleasures—which previously were all that would wake us from our sensory torpor. The more the body is absent to the world, the more intensity is expected and sought after in order to free the ensuing tension. This absence reaches its culmination in sadomasochistic practices, which attempt to bring an abandoned body into a state of tremoring vibration.

A yogini or yogi allows all sensory systems to be in constant tremoring. Satisfaction is thus continuous and deep. It opens into continuous joy.

According to the different temperatures it experiences, the contacts it makes, the bodies it approaches or avoids, the skin will provide us with thousands of important pieces of information with which we can choose to communicate.

One of the great discoveries of presence is that we can have total trust in the body. It knows. It is marvelously capable of providing us with an immediate response to most situations in which a choice is required. Unfortunately, we do not recognize this ability of the body; very often our reflections trouble us and push us to make decisions that go against the body. When this happens, we often say, "I knew"—which means, "My body knew." The more we learn to trust our body totally, the more we will discover that it naturally guides us to a joyous spontaneity.

A day lived in partial consciousness of the breath and of the sense of touch is a day which tends more and more toward plenitude and toward the deep satisfaction of our longings, in proportion to the development of this consciousness.

# 9

## The Heart of Reality

We often succeed—and I have done this with a certain artistry—in following a spiritual path without this path transforming our daily reality. We become interested, we listen to the teachings, we adhere, become Buddhist, tantrika, Vedantin, Sufi, whatever. This simple change soothes us into a pleasant state but does not always lead us back to the everyday.

Instead we follow our chosen spiritual path, discover its mysteries, have moments of beautiful depth when we are in the company of our peers or when we spend time with our master. We read passionately, we take in a new philosophy, we devote some time each day to meditation and other practices. A little altar with a little image of Shiva or the Buddha along with a photo of our master reminds us of this new life. Every day we offer flowers and incense—all without undergoing any radical transformation of our ordinary life.

This duality comes from the fact that we are pursuing a spiritual fantasy—however refined it may be—without engaging ourselves totally in the quest. We are surprised, then, that our reactions are the same, that our actions reveal not a trace of our meditation, that our vows, the precepts that we observe, are simple safety nets incapable of transforming us. In fact, we do not want to communicate deeply with the reality of what we are; we prefer to develop a little island of devotion to which we can take escape from time to time.

The Kashmiri masters understood well this process of absence to reality in the spiritual quest. Over the course of a few thousand years, they considered all angles of this issue and invented a simple and refined practice whereby human beings choose as their domain of practice the whole of day-to-day reality within society, without either renouncing or separating themselves from anything whatsoever, but instead simply allowing consciousness to emerge in each act of life.

Every day, with a mischievous gleam in her eye, my master Devi would ask me what the practice was changing in my daily life. Her objective was to help me realize whether, from the moment I opened my eyes until the moment I closed them again, I was present to my manner of walking and breathing; to each instant of life; to the harmony of each contact, each gesture, each sensation, each emotion, each thought. For Devi the entire domain of reality had to be laid seige to by allowing consciousness to engulf it.

From the beginning of my time with her, Devi made me notice every instant of absence from the world, every abrupt or unrefined movement or action, every automatism. Her teaching was centered upon an easeful but continual presence to the world. When she spoke to me of philosophy, she always brought the ideas back to the reality of life and to constant practice.

For Devi, a person who aspires to spirituality is a person who allows all actions or movements that connect her to the world to circulate freely and unendingly, as much on the interior level of sensations, emotions, and thoughts as on the level of action. She would say that a single instant of total presence was worth the reading of all the texts, all the poets, all the philosophers. Devi was a great *sahajiya*, a totally spontaneous, awakened being.

At first this insistence was unpleasant for me because it was an affront to my spiritual dream. I felt like a sort of chaotically gesturing paralytic whose automatisms were so deep that I rarely emerged from them. I could not physically escape Devi's presence day or night, so it was impossible for me to get away from this continual consciousness.

I would have preferred to have to practice a ritual, recite mantras, concentrate on *yantras*, do prostrations, meditate for hours on end like I had done while practicing Vipassana in Thailand. But Devi was not there to give me what I expected; she was there to help me liberate myself within the ordinariness of the everyday, and this was the revolution of my life.

There was no ritual other than to breathe, walk, bathe in the icy water of the waterfall; to look at the earth, the lichens, the trees, the leaves, common objects; to enter deeply into contact with life, reality. "Adhere deeply to reality with the heart of your being; there is nothing else to look for!" she would say.

This path, in the beginning, lacks notably in the exotic, the magical, the extraordinary. Nothing spectacular, nothing shifting in terms of exterior energy, but only inner stirrings! Everything is a question of being in tune. The Kashmiris, great lovers of music, like to compare the yogini or the yogi to the *sarangi*, a stringed instrument, the tuning of which is a particularly intricate and long process because of its number of interrelated strings.

I had loved quivering to the sound of Tibetan music, every night, in Sonada, at the Kalou Rinpoche's monastery. I had been transported to other realms by my master and by those I had sat close to, thanks to him. I had vibrated to the practices in the warm and relaxed, humorous and rigorous Tibetan atmosphere. With Devi, nothing happened. We would draw water, prepare our frugal meals, remain seated in silence; she would give me the teachings; we would walk, enjoy the sun, have fun in a relaxed way—but with presence.

I tried simply to touch life, to really experience it, under the searching, generous, and intense gaze of this woman who seemed to me like a light scented breeze, like an unshakable rock, like a capricious brook following the meanderings of reality moment after moment, and sometimes also like an incandescent wave that would submerge me with violence.

The smallest thing would fill her with wonder. Her ecstasy was continually fed by the slightest modification of things. In her there was no intentionality at all, simply an immediate and unfailing enjoyment of each moment. In comparison and despite my sensual nature, I had the impression of being totally cut off from the world. Her steadfast joy, her brilliant gaze, her continual tremoring gave the impression that she was making love with the tiniest particles of the universe.

Little by little she initiated me to this nonpostural yoga of presence that emerges from consciousness. For tantrikas, consciousness does not proceed from activity; on the contrary, it is activity that flows from consciousness. Thus, our senses do not perceive an outer object in order to pull it inward, toward the perceiver; on the contrary, it is consciousness that emerges, goes out and touches the world, and in this way brings back the whole manifestation to its source. This explains why the tantrikas of the various schools, the practitioners of *dzogchen*, Mahamudra, and Ch'an, insist on presence to reality. Without it there is no consciousness, and without consciousness a practice bears no fruit.

# 10

# *The Source of Consciousness*

*A*ll these teachings begin with this very simple observation: There is only consciousness. The various yogas are not means to reach this consciousness. Abhinavagupta, the tenth-century Tantric philosopher and one of India's greatest thinkers, says in his monumental work *Tantraloka* ("light on the Tantras"): "All that is proscribed, all that is upheld, the yogas based on such limbs as the control of breath or other things, all that is false."[12]

In thus freeing themselves from the different types of yoga, the Tantric masters wanted to point toward this solely existing consciousness and, for them, attention to reality is the simplest and most direct way for consciousness to manifest itself continuously. Only reason is retained because it allows "a larger, all-encompassing, consciousness of great acuteness which goes on continually interiorising itself more and more," says Abhinavagupta in the same text.[13]

As can be seen, this constant recourse to the source of existence exonerates the tantrika from all adherence to any moral or ethical precepts. The tantrika rejects all interdictions, all exterior and progressive quests that involve the intervention of ritualistic forms or beliefs or dogmas and even metaphysics, which has no effect on the practical level. This is also one of the fundamental teachings of the Buddha, who never responded to these types of questions.

There is neither transcendence nor purification. The masters define *purity* as "all that is lived with consciousness," and *impurity* as "all that is lived with automatism and non-presence." Consciousness replaces everything, and without it there is no spirituality.

In order to arrive at this profound consciousness, it is indispensable that our instrument, the body, be perfectly in tune, and this is where the whole issue of our sensorality comes in. What would be the worth of a body whose marvelous functionings were not operating? How would consciousness spherically unfold itself within a frozen form not tending toward natural fluidity?

The first step is therefore to restore these functions, to regain our taste for life, our capacity to perceive the world with the continual wonder of a child. It will be easily understood that this can happen only within a larger, all-encompassing acceptance of what we really are. Such a task becomes impossible if we imagine ourselves otherwise, if we idealize ourselves, if we erase a part of our personality whenever we discover within ourselves territories unworthy of the path.

This self-acceptance is a very delicate process because it implies deep contact with our shadow side, all our opacity, and all the secret sources buried in the deepest part of us. Entering wholly onto this path is the only way to avoid later crashing into what we would have chopped off of ourselves—which would have grown considerably in the darkness. Everything that we abandon in the false dream of conforming to a system is precisely what will subsequently come along and block our path.

This approach restores free will, since submission to a religious authority or to one of its messengers thus no longer exists. There is no one who could bring us revelation or serve as intermediator between the divine realms and our thirst for plenitude; if there were, these would not be present within us. Everything tremors interiorly, and we possess the whole of the means to gain access to this world. We are the divine, we are the temple, we are the worshiper. Total and immaculate consciousness has always been within us; nothing and no one can give it to us or alter its scintillating quality.

Thus it is no longer a question of cutting off the senses, desires, and passions; on the contrary, it is a question of mounting these high-spirited, steedlike messengers in full consciousness so that they may carry us rapidly to a continuous presence to the world. This all-encompassing, larger conception of the profound dignity of the human being is often misunderstood. Certain people imagine that it refers to permissiveness, and in allowing themselves to follow their egoist inclinations they bind themselves increasingly in suffering and absence. This is the battle of impulsiveness against spontaneity. Impulsiveness is brutal and destructive, because it is unconscious of the other and of the world. Spontaneity is full of grace, for it is granted immediately through consciousness to the reality of the environment.

> Our desires are powerless if they do not dip into the vibrating Reality. It is true that one can realise nothing without desire; thus must one plunge desire into the efficiency of Spanda [divine, inner tremoring vibration]. If one puts all his energy into a single desire, if one goes all the way with his impulse-force, then one will join again the divine energy of desire.[14]

"The body immediately confers perfection, that is, certainty with regard to the true nature of things . . . thanks to the contact with the power of the Self," says Abhinavagupta.[15]

But how to desire without suffering? How to surrender to passion without experiencing destruction? Why do almost all the spiritual paths prohibit sensorality, desire, and passion? Why cut off a part of human potential in order to find plenitude? What kind of plenitude would it be if it did not include the totality of the human?

Here again, the Tantric masters have fully and completely rejected all prejudices. They have considered with both awareness and full consciousness all the jolts that pass through a human being and, rather than deny these lively and intense forces, they have forgotten what humans claim to know about their passions and instead examined them directly, with naked attention.

In this way, over the course of the thousands of years during which the transmission of Tantrism has taken place, they have come to some surprising and totally innovative conclusions on sensorality, desires, and passions.

## II

*Savoring the World*

*I*n the same proportion that we find our home in the breath, and as our tactile sensorality is developed, we will discover that our savoring of the world becomes richer. Our tongue is sensitive to the molecules that come into contact with it. This sense functions in close connection with the olfactory sense.

Tantric yoga proposes that we change our perspective on desire in order to improve our perceptions and our sense of taste. While drinking a glass of water, for example, if we believe that this water desires us, we will have an experience of consciousness; we will feel the water penetrate into us and cross through us. Everything we taste can then bring us the fundamental experience of union with the elements. Stanza 72 of the *Vijnanabhairava Tantra* addresses this experience directly: "At the time of euphoria and expansion caused by delicate foods and drinks, be total in this delight, and through it, taste supreme bliss."[16] This constant attention to the savor of things leads us directly to the experience of the divine through full consciousness. It removes all distance between

44

the world and us, restoring from moment to moment our active participation in life.

⟜

*I become aware of everything that touches my tongue, my palate, my mouth. I open myself to sensation, to the taste of things and people.*

*My lips and my tongue are among the most sensitive areas of my body. I use them in full consciousness to come into contact with the world. Like a child, I make a game of putting into my mouth whatever I am drawn to, and I rediscover forgotten tastes.*

*I allow my body to come into a state of vibration through fine foods.*

*I benefit from the sharing of a meal in order to let all my senses open to the presence of the other.*

⟜

## 12

# Desire and Its Object

$\mathcal{D}$esire is one of our life forces. To deny desire or to want to cut it off is to deprive ourselves of an incomparable dynamic; it is to head toward becoming dried up and drained of life, the mark of so many of the "religious." *Religious* means "bound." What better bond than desire? The Kashmiri masters recognized this power, and their questioning was not concerned with desire in and of itself, indispensable, but with the bonds between desire and its object.

If everything proceeds from consciousness, then no one action is more worthy than any other. The desire for God is a desire; the desire to renounce desire is itself a desire. It is therefore impossible to follow a spiritual or mystical path while eradicating desire. For tantrikas, desire is the mark of the endless creativity of consciousness. In cutting it off, we cut off an important part of our consciousness.

Stanza 105 of the *Vijnanabhairava Tantra*,[17] one of the most ancient Tantric texts and the source of all nonpostural yoga, describes this choice position: "Desire exists in you as in everything. Realize that it also resides in objects and in all that the mind can grasp. Then, in discovering the universality of desire, enter its radiant space."[18]

For tantrikas, desire is the very movement, the very nature, of the universe itself. In order not to have to cut it off, they considered it in its absolute form and asked themselves the question: "What do we really desire?" We can readily believe—and this corresponds in general to our fragmented experience of the world—that we desire to possess people or objects. Hence, we go through the world as predators, seeking to appropriate for ourselves everything our desire can touch. After a short time, we realize that we are dissatisfied, and this mechanism of truncated desire pushes us unceasingly to desire more objects, in an endless cycle that eventually gives way to frustration.

"What if *desire* were to desire something other than objects?" the Tantric masters then wondered. If desire were simply the incandescence that gives us the feeling of being alive, were intensity, were the tremoring vibration that carries us, then it would be absurd to allow it to be consumed by objects and to lose it once we possess the object or realize we cannot attain it. This profound movement is life itself, and this tremoring is the one that all yoginis and yogis experience, precisely because they remain in the incandescence of desire without rendering it dependent upon the object. In this instant, objects are seen as maintaining incandescence and not as reducing it.

In the Tantric *sadhana* there is a particular practice, connected to the stanza cited above, wherein the yogi sees the world as desire. Everything—a leaf falling from a tree, the sky, the snow, the water he drinks, his food—desires him. In this way he enters into an extremely subtle and refined relationship with objects. We do not touch in the same way a teacup that desires us, we do not look in the same way at a tree that desires us, because each contact with reality becomes a celebration of the universality of desire. Fixation on a single object thus ceases to exist.

"You miss one person and the whole world seems empty of people": Lamartine's verse well expresses this kind of absence to the world in which we become completely unbalanced by a desire centered on one single person, on one single thing that obsesses us to the point of masking the world from us.

The obstacle to our continual satisfaction is that we reduce our desire instead of allowing it to blossom out over all objects. A reduced desire blocks the fluidity of consciousness, sensations, thoughts, and emotions. When a single object takes an exclusive place in our mind, when our being reaches toward this object in a sort of contracted tension, movement ceases within us and suffering finds its home in us.

On the other hand, when our desire occupies all of space the absence of one object goes totally unnoticed, because the flow of our awareness remains free to come into contact with thousands of others. This is the way tantrikas live: in constant presence to the whole of reality. They are thus incessantly showered by the world's infinite variety. They no longer have to seize, to stifle, objects; they leave them free, and the contact they have with the world is of such richness that lack, frustration, or solitude never comes and finds its home in them.

The incandescence of the desire that burns from its own indistinguishable fire is what makes the tantrikas' gaze shine so brilliantly, what makes them perpetually in love with reality, what makes them so alive, so tremoring, whereas, all the while, they consume nothing, or almost.

In Devi's company I perceived the supremacy of her desire, which included all objects, while mine spent its time exhausting itself by isolating one object after another, absent to multiplicity. For us, everything is consciousness, and everything that manifests itself leads us unceasingly back to consciousness. The senses thus become a marvelous palette that we open to the world, painting it with a thousand colors so that reality unceasingly leads us back to our own Self in a loving, fluid, and unfettered dynamic.

# 13

## The Supreme Reality

The worlds are not split in two. The absolute is at the very heart of reality. Everything is vibrating, everything is real. We do not believe that phenomena are illusory, and we come very close to Ch'an Buddhism in this vision of the reality of the world as consciousness void of a separate reality. Everything is interconnected; everything is at the same time image and reflection.

That we talk about the Self brings us close to certain Buddhist schools like the Yogacara of Asanga, who speaks of the Great Self. The tantrikas furthermore say that one of the names of Shiva is the Great Void or the Great Spatiality, which contains the whole world, all forms, all thoughts, and all emotions like the Void of certain historic masters of Buddhism. Notes the Sixth Patriarch of Ch'an:

> *Maha* means "great." The capacity of the mind is vast and great like empty space, and has no boundaries. . . .
>
> Good Knowing Advisors, do not listen to my explanation of emptiness and then become attached to empti-

ness. If you sit still with an empty mind you will become attached to undifferentiated emptiness. . . .

Good Knowing Advisors, the emptiness of the universe is able to contain the forms and shapes of the ten thousand things: the sun, the moon, and stars; the mountains, rivers, and the great earth; the fountains, springs, streams, torrents, grasses, trees, thickets and forests; good and bad people, good and bad dharmas, the heavens and the hells, all the great seas, Sumeru* and all mountains— all are contained within emptiness.[19]

What is it that comes to block us in this spherical unfolding of the senses, in the fire of desire, and causes our experience of reality to be unceasingly torn between pleasure and suffering? What keeps us from having a taste of continual presence of desire?

Here again the Kashmiri masters return to the source, consciousness. We are capable of living the reality of the world directly, without the mental faculties incessantly deferring this enjoyment by coming in to comment on it, judge it, ensconce it in differentiation.

The naked awareness that allows sensations, emotions, and thoughts not to become fixed or frozen within us is what we can contact during contemplation or meditation. Everything starts by the examination of what is—that is, our trouble, our difficulty, in perceiving all things in the moment. Presence to agitation is the opening toward peacefulness. We never try to change, to adopt a new way of behaving; instead, we try only to allow our awareness to descend toward what is really happening within us. We will notice that this presence

---

* Patriarch's note: *Sumeru* is the central mountain of every world system, translated into Chinese as *miao kao*, "wonderfully high."

is sufficient for putting an end to whatever is blocking the fluidity of life.

Thus, in this peace and silence we see clearly our troubled and confused reality. We grasp the fact that this trouble is linked to the dynamic of our agitated mind, which incessantly judges, classifies, accepts, rejects, flees, or attempts to grab hold of events. A calm awareness will cause us to come into contact with a different reality: that the body has an unlimited capacity for being in tune with the world with extraordinary precision, grace, and spontaneity—if we stop blocking it by our thought, which always defers to doubt, to others' views, to guilt, to the fundamental fear of being nothing.

In the *Hevajra Tantra*, we read:

> In the absence of the body where is there bliss, for without the body it is not possible to speak about bliss. The world is pervaded by bliss, the world and bliss being mutually dependent.
>
> Just as smell in the flower does not exist in the absence of the flower, similarly bliss is not experienced in the absence of form and other qualities.
>
> I am existence as well as not existence. I am the Enlightened One for I am enlightened regarding the true nature of things. But those fools who are affected by dullness do not know me.[20]

When we lose the whole idea of the impurity of the body, then this bliss finds its home in us. Shiva proclaims:

> Oh Devi, some people claim, "The body is made up of impurities such as germs, worms, faeces, urine, phlegm, blood, flesh, skin, and so on. How can we offer such a body to the Guru?" With thoughts like these, they don't make an offering.

This is not right. The body in which the Guru and the Self dwell can only be considered pure. There should never be any feeling of impurity about offering the body.

*Seventy-two thousand channels*
*threading through five sheaths,*
*here the Self ever makes its home.*
*Muktananda, the wise ones see it*
*as the temple of the Lord.*[21]

# 14

## Naked Awareness

The ego is, above all, separation. When desire does not unfold itself toward the ego, it spontaneously immerses itself in consciousness. In this way, the same thing that ties people conditioned by the ego liberates the tantrika, and desire blossoms into pure love. Obstruction then ceases to exist. If, in presence, we can descend to the deepest in ourselves, we see clearly that there is no ego, no differentiation, and therefore no duality. At this moment fear is no longer present and we can at last, for brief moments, experience the state of the *sahajiya*—"awakened adept of spontaneity"—which is how the tantrikas define themselves, whether Shaivists or Buddhists. Chinul, the twelfth-century Korean Ch'an master, expresses this freedom magnificently in his treatise *Secrets of Cultivating the Mind:*

> Thus for adepts the principle of equally maintaining concentration and insight is not a matter of effort; it is spontaneous and effortless, with no more particular time frame. When seeing and hearing, they are just so; when

defecating and urinating, they are just so; when convers-
ing with people, they are just so; whatever they are doing, walking, standing, sitting, reclining, speaking, silent,
rejoicing, raging, at all times and in everything they are
thus, like empty boats riding the waves, going along with
the high and the low, like a river winding through the
mountains, curving at curves and straight at straits, without minding any state of mind, buoyantly going along
with nature today, going along with nature buoyantly
tomorrow, adapting to all circumstances without inhibition or impediment, neither stopping nor fostering good
or evil, simple and straightforward, without artificiality,
perception normal.[22]

For tantrikas, the ego itself has no core other than consciousness. Once the ego lets go a little, relaxes, eases up, its
fundamentally absolute nature frees itself. The ego therefore
is not to be cut off, any more than is everything else that makes
a human being. Grasping its original immaculate and spatial
nature is enough.

Stanza 146 of the *Vijnanabhairava Tantra* offers this very
beautiful definition of meditation: "A stable and character-less
mind, there is true contemplation. . . ,"[23] while the *sahajiyas*
talk about "consciousness as stability, ease, repose, quiescence."
When the mind finds itself calmed in this way, it is at last able
to reflect reality as it is and not as we would like it to be. This
incessant reorchestrating of our mind, which makes every effort to see the world as it imagines it, tires us and causes us
suffering. A peaceful mind realizes that it has the ability to
grasp everything instantaneously. It no longer has to "stock-
pile" the materials of reality in order to deal with them later. It
sees things directly, without projection and without judgment,
in all their evidence and obviousness, in their naked reality.

Our desires, our passions, and our senses then cease to be a problem for us. All that they reap in the dailiness of our lives bring us bliss, and we finally perceive that life can be fully lived.

The whole difficulty of the spontaneity for which the tantrika longs, whether Shaivist or Buddhist, is to succeed in seizing the moment with the same lively agility with which one would seize a venomous snake. Hesitation can be fatal.

When reality presents itself to us, we can seize it only in instantaneousness. If we succeed in this spontaneous act, we live upstream of differentiating thought *(vikalpa)*, and each thing presents itself in its naked reality. If we arrive too late, the mental flow will have already introduced a separation between us and the world, and we will have to wait for the next opportunity to be spontaneous. The yogini and the yogi have the intense agility of a tiger. The moment does not escape them because they have returned desire and the activity of the senses to their absolute nature. There is therefore no repression, no avoidance, no transcendence. Asanga, citing the Buddha, says this well: "No outcome for attraction other than attraction and the same goes for aversion and distraction, for nothing is independent of the essence of things."[24]

This specifically Tantric yoga is simple yet not easily accessible, because it is tied to ordinary experience. Says Saraha:

> *By means of that same essence by which one is born, lives and*
> *    dies,*
> *By means of that one gains the highest bliss.*[25]

To keep oneself sharp, lively and quick, spontaneous, and alert to the instant when things arise is considered the Mahayoga by the tantrikas because the success of this small miracle of presence dispenses with all expedients, all techniques, all spiritual practices, all the specific yogas. It is supreme nonpractice, since in the lightning flash of the moment all becoming and all progression on the spiritual path are annihilated. This is the quintessence of Tantrism, of Ch'an, of *dzogchen*, the Great Seal, or Mahamudra (as the Tibetans and Kashmiris call it). Saraha expresses this in a magnificent verse of his *Dohakosa:*

> *O know this truth,*
> *That neither at home nor in the forest does enlightenment*
>   *dwell.*
> *Be free from prevarication*
> *In the self [essential]-nature of immaculate thought*
>   *[consciousness]!*[26]

This "immaculate thought" or "immaculate consciousness" is total freedom. To reach it, tantrikas do not merely talk about it. They teach how to get there, and that is the heart of Tantra.

## 15

*Sounds of Life*

The sense of hearing is a marvelous revealer of space. It is enough to close the eyes, to let this sense expand, to perceive that it is in tune with the greatest subtlety. If we let ourselves be carried by the wave of our perception, we can discover farther and farther horizons, to the limit of silence.

The quivering vibration of people's voices opens us to awareness. Music enchants us and causes us to come into contact with our deepest emotions. It allows us to explore a choice realm where a peaceful mind allows itself to be won over by all-encompassing intuition. Music permits the body to move and regain its fundamental freedom of expression through dance. We hear with our whole body; we directly perceive the vibrations of certain instruments, which touch us like a caress or penetrate us more deeply.

We love to "listen to silence" or to the infinitesimal noises that inhabit the silent universe. These tremoring sounds calm us and make us sensitive to subtlety, to the opening of our being to the world.

"At the moment where your attention awakens through sensory organs, enter the spatiality of your own heart," advises the *Vijnanabhairava Tantra*, stanza 136.[27]

*I open my sensitivity to the arising and passing of sounds that lead me back to my own plenitude.*

*I let my body respond to sounds, to music. I let my instrument be permanently in tune so that I can take part in the cosmic concert.*

*I abandon myself, surrender, to the sound of my own breath, to someone else's. I communicate with the sound of the breath, which brings me space and peace.*

*I listen to others with total presence. My whole body listens and, beyond language, I hear what these bodies are telling me.*

## 16

## The Essence of Satisfaction

Stanza 74 of the *Vijnanabhairava Tantra* tells us clearly: "Wherever you find satisfaction, the very essence of bliss will be revealed to you if you remain in this place without wavering."[28] This is *saktopaya*. To practice this stanza and live the sensations that a tantrika knows, experience them yourself. Each day, according to your sensitivity and your mood, choose to enter into total communication with the objects of your desire or, more simply, with the states that spontaneously present themselves and that harbor the power to bring you a kind of satisfaction you no doubt underestimate.

As soon as you awaken, enter into consciousness in your body, considered the temple of the divine. Observe physiological changes (sensation of breath, of tensions, of the heartbeat, of blood flow, of the diaphragm, of the intestines, and so on); note the start of mental activity, the flow of sensations and emotions. Do this for twenty or thirty seconds, like an extended interior cinematic moving shot of the inner landscapes, zooming forward and back; then, consciously, withdraw from this awareness and return to your habitual manner of doing things—that is, to automatic pilot.

A little later, while getting up, for example, bring the same naked and nonjudgmental attention to the movements of your body and muscles. After a few seconds, withdraw your attention. A little later, as you walk barefoot on the floor, for four or five steps be present to your feet, to your movements, to your sensations, then come back to the habitual course of things. Be present to a few sips of whatever you are drinking and return to automatism. Next, in the time it takes to butter a slice of bread, do this same back-and-forthing with presence. When you taste your piece of bread, return once more to presence and then release.

When you leave the house, give a few seconds of your attention to the sky then, after a break, to the movements of your body. Continue in this manner, consciously entering into and then emerging from presence. Be present to a face, to a look, to thirty seconds of a conversation in which you listen to the whole person who is speaking to you and not only to her words. If you succeed with this light, open awareness, in the spirit of a game, free from all religious or spiritual ideas, you will make, starting from the first day, a series of major discoveries that will help you to be totally alive.

You do not need to be Buddhist or tantrika; you do not even need to be interested in spirituality. It is a matter of but one reality: your desire to be in the world, totally, without inhibition, without fear, without anxiety. The desire to be wholly available to life suffices. You do not have to be involved in, or to practice, or to believe anything whatsoever. The ultimate things present themselves in such a simple way that it is enough to experience them by yourself.

What passionate things will you discover? You will see that each time you succeed in seizing life in its immediacy, your breath will relax harmoniously. This sensation will bring you deep pleasure; you will feel it to the very innermost part of your head. Ten seconds of spontaneous breathing, gentle and deep, is enough to release a kind of vibrating stream of warmth into your brain and sometimes into your whole body.

Next, you will discover that true presence brings you pleasure incommensurate with events. The most banal thing—a cup of tea, a few steps, opening a door, a glance at the sky—can be enough to make you happy during the time you are present and well after.

You will discover that if you can find such pleasure in presence, then your joy no longer depends on exceptional circumstances waited for in a state of neurotic tension but on simple reality, as it presents itself to you from moment to moment. In this way you will gain immense autonomy from the intense pleasures that you once needed in order to be satisfied.

It will very quickly follow from there that your quest and your expectations will no longer be focused on hypothetical or uncertain objects but on whatever your experience reveals to you about everyday ordinariness.

You will discover that nothing or no one can take this pleasure away from you. Again, your independence will increase.

You will discover that your body and your mind love this communication so much that they will unite and ask you for more of it. The habitual schism between the body and mind will progressively subside.

You will perceive that with presence to the world, there is no ego, and therefore no separation, no duality. The panic about being nothing that swells in the back of your mind will then subside, leaving room for you to experience that to be nothing is to enter into totality, and that in this naked awareness you are the world. Your body will regain a feeling of plenitude and calm. Even if, in the beginning, this lasts only three minutes a day, it will change your life to an extent that you cannot imagine.

This attention to life as I have just presented it to you is simple because it totally coincides with the rapid flow of the mind. It does not require reserving extensive stretches of time for practice; it does not require adhering to any principles or buying any materials, and you can do it anywhere. This is what in Kashmiri Tantra are called the micropractices. Nothing is more efficient, nothing is simpler, nothing is more profound. These are not preliminaries: This is the whole practice of Tantra in all its splendor. There is no higher goal.

What will happen if you decide to practice this yoga sixty times a day for fifteen seconds? You will spend fifteen minutes a day "being." At first three or four minutes will suffice. You will increase not the duration of the practices but their number. This will be a kind of game that you can practice without anyone knowing. You will not even need to claim to be Buddhist, Sufi, or tantrika, but simply human, the most natural in the world. People around you will be much more deeply affected by your presence than by your speeches and your spiritual theories. Presence is contagious. People will ask you if you are in love, and you will spontaneously answer "yes" without quite knowing with whom or with what you are in love. It is this continuous feeling that will henceforth guide your life.

If this practice speaks to you and if you persevere for a few weeks, or a few months, you will discover that there is no longer a "practice" but quite simply pleasure, an incomparable tremoring thrill for life. At that moment you will contact the Tantric secret, and you will naturally journey toward a more and more steady pleasure of presence, because this is the profound meaning of life. Little by little you will realize that what is hidden behind the most inaccessible treatises, the most sophisticated philosophy, the most secret practices, is simply this.

You will then approach the source from which all the spiritual and mystical paths spring and, in unceasingly deepening your naked presence to the world, you will experience what we call awakening.

# 17

## Sensorality and Consciousness

*I*t has often been said that the historical masters of Kashmiri Shaivism were closer to the Sufis than to the Buddhists. It is true that in the Kashmiri texts there are little hints of humor aimed at the Buddhists, but there was also a fascination for certain Buddhists schools to which the Kashmiris felt very close. The Yogacara school, founded by Asanga and Vasubandhu, two brothers who lived in the fourth century, profoundly influenced the tantrikas. Ch'an, influenced by this same school and by the *Lankavatara Sutra*, most likely written toward the fifth century, is also very close.

Abhinavagupta, the tenth-century Tantric philosopher, a grammarian, poet, musician, and man of encyclopedic knowledge, pays homage in his works to twenty of his masters. He did not limit himself to Shivaism, but equally followed the Jain masters or Buddhists of the Yogacara school. The Tantric tradition, well rooted in Kashmir, of searching for knowledge wherever it appears is fairly exceptional. In traditional India people would more likely be inclined to follow just one school and one master. Perhaps because of its geographical location, Kashmir, a place of communication and passage, was as open to Islam as to China, Tibet, and India. The merchants of the silk trade route liked to go to Kashmir to rest or holiday; the original Tibetan masters went there to seek the teachings and to be near the Siddhas (perfected or realized beings) and the Tantric yoginis. Chinese monks and pilgrims made Kashmir one of their prime access routes to India, and in all the written travel accounts, this region has always been likened to a sort of paradise. In this atmosphere of intense communication, Shivaism profoundly influenced Buddhism and in return drank from the Yogacara source, especially in the conception of the eight consciousnesses.

In order to understand truly the place of the senses, desire, and passion in Tantrism, it is indispensable to grasp how Asanga saw consciousness. His vision, of unequaled depth and refinement, permits us to grasp in all its complex subtlety the senses' spherical unfolding out of consciousness and the return of this flow into the spatial Self, as he describes it. Upon this concept of consciousness hinges the whole process of knowing.

Yogacara and tantrika recognize eight consciousnesses:

THE FIVE SENSORY CONSCIOUSNESSES

1. Visual consciousness
2. Olfactory consciousness
3. Feeling or tactile consciousness
4. Gustative consciousness
5. Auditory consciousness

THE TWO MENTAL CONSCIOUSNESSES

6. Consciousness tied to the ego, and therefore to duality *(manas)*

7. Nondual consciousness, which directly centralizes
the sensations *(manovijñâna)*

## INNERMOST CONSCIOUSNESS OR UNCONSCIOUS (DIVIDED INTO TWO)

8a. Unconscious polluted by its ties to the ego
*(âlayavijñâna)*
8b. Immaculate consciousness, core of being
*(amalavijñâna)*

This division has the advantage of making all mental and sensory activity absolutely clear. It shows how yoginis and yogis—Buddhists, tantrikas, or Tantric Buddhists—perceive reality and how the whole of reality always comes back toward immaculate consciousness in an uninterrupted cycle. This division brings to light the manner in which consciousness becomes troubled, how it accumulates slag in the unconscious, and the way in which consciousness can liberate itself from these absorbed marks of the past that permeate it. This division shows how the *I* and the ego are formed and how they oppose the absolute clarity of the *I Am* freed from all ties to the narrow views of the *I*. How, finally, the game of perception either feeds the unconscious, adding to our confusion or trouble and annihilating our chances of perceiving reality in its essence, or on the other hand shrouds each sensation in the enjoyment of original spontaneous freedom.

For Asanga, the sixth, mental consciousness *(manas)* is the site of all our troubles and anxieties. It is through its identification with the *I* that it creates the ego, sustains it, and reinforces it with each sensation. This is where duality is born, where the world splits into subject and object. This is where observer and observed exist; where differentiating discourse, which will incessantly come along and obscure our understanding of reality, is raised. Linked to memory, this consciousness also allows us to function remarkably, but when absolute reality takes it by seige, it is the cause of all our ego-related errors of interpretation of reality. This is why "objective" consciousness, so prized by Western cultures, is for the Kashmiris and the Buddhists much less profound than what they call "pure subjectivity," which is in fact related to the seventh, mental consciousness. In the yogini and the yogi it is certainly present, but its easeful quality prevents any clashes with the ego's displays. It functions admirably without leading the universe back toward the *I*. It allows the liberated person to live in action.

The seventh, mental consciousness *(manovijñāna)* could be compared with a computer that would centralize all perceptions and assure communication without elevating the ego, which would maintain the illusion of being a separate entity from the world. In the universe of the seventh consciousness the senses communicate to us their continual harvest with absolute freshness, unmarred by any of the absorbed influences or refuse of the past. There is no more duality, no more distance between the world and the yogi or yogini, who as a result marvels at all that surfaces in this consciousness. It is this consciousness that is operating in each instant of total presence to the reality of a sensation, a thought, or an emotion. The play of this centralizing and neutral consciousness does not add anything to a perception; it does not compare it with others, or name, label, devalue, or exaggerate anything that presents itself to us. You can have this experience of naked, unrepeatable sensation by practicing for a few weeks the yoga of presence presented in chapter 16, and thereby come into contact with your own unique reality.

## 18

## The Interaction of the Eight Consciousnesses

The manner in which the play of the sixth and seventh consciousnesses liberates or enslaves appears even more clearly when we examine their connection with the eighth consciousness, or innermost consciousness. It is remarkable to see that, from the first centuries of the Common Era, these thinkers and philosophers had not only defined the unconscious *(âlayavijñâna)* but had also descended to an even subtler level of consciousness, which they call immaculate consciousness *(amalavijñâna)*. It is this latter consciousness that the *Lankavatara Sutra* identifies with *tathagatagharba*—embryo or womb, one's own or proper nature, or Buddha state—and that the Kashmiri Shaivists link to Parama Shiva, absolute consciousness or Self.

But the Ch'an and Tantric thinkers go farther still. In effect, dividing consciousness into eight categories would constitute a return to separation; this splitting can only be realized by the sixth consciousness, differentiation. It is important, therefore, to reunite what thought has divided into a constant striving toward the absolute, and this is the experience of the yogi and yogini. The masters of Yogacara, Ch'an, and Tantrism are thus saying what we read in the *Lankavatara Sutra*: "The Tathagatagharba known as *Alayavijñana* evolves together with the seven *Vijñanas* [consciousnesses]."[29] All experience, all sensorality, is hence reintegrated with the absolute, which forms out of or from them the underlying layer or core. There is, then, no longer any reason for the tantrika, the Ch'an adept, or the Yogacara school adept to flee the experience of the senses or that of reality in order to reach the absolute. On the contrary, each contact will reveal, to the yogi or yogini detached from the ego, absolute consciousness.

The Buddha said this clearly: "I teach Reality. . . . That is the inner realm truly taught by the Masters." And in the same sutra:

> The Gharba of the Tathagatas [pure Buddha nature] is indeed *united* with the seven *Vijñânas*; when this is adhered to, there arises duality, but when rightly understood, duality ceases.[30]

Ma-tsu, the sublime Ch'an master of the eighth century, borrowing from the *Lankavatara Sutra* transmitted by Bodhidharma, declared: "There is not a trace of the absolute outside of reality."[31] And Utpaladevi, poet, philosopher and Tantric master of the tenth century, would go on to sing:

> *Having seen the world as consisting of your nature*
> *And having realized the pleasure*
> *Of your non-dual form,*
> *Still may I never part*
> *With the enjoyment of the spirit of devotion.*
>
> *Whatever is not,*
> *Let that be nothing to me.*

*Whatever is,*
*Let that be something to me.*
*In this way may it be*
*That you be found and worshipped by me*
*In all states.*[32]

# 19

## The Power
## of the Senses

$\mathcal{B}$haskara, another great Kashmiri master of the Vasugupta lineage, writes in his commentary on the *Shiva Sutras:* "The senses have the power to make this new creation emerge, as experience proves, because they are sustained by the inborn power of the consciousness. It is thus because the power of the senses comes from the absorbing force existing in the Self." Bhaskara sees in the activity of the senses the authentic foundation of existence.

For the person who does not communicate with reality, everything is illusory. Everything takes on a static form that the ego fixes and weighs down. From this illusion, which egoistic people call reality, are born suffering, solitude, separation. All these impressions will get dumped into the unconscious, or the obscure part of innermost unconsciousness, and all these reverberations will set the stage for the never-ending cycle of the person enchained within the spheres of illusion, dependence, and unhappiness.

How to escape this cycle? By total ease and presence to reality, according to the teachings of Yogacara Buddhism,

Ch'an, *dzogchen*, and Tantrism. Consciousness, says Asanga, is "hindered by the view of the 'I': from there comes its agitated and powerless tension. This can be remedied by stabilizing consciousness in the inner world, which amounts to re-establishing consciousness in consciousness itself."[33]

It is therefore solely by letting go of what Asanga calls "the mass of tension" of differentiating thought that we can attain a peaceful state of the body-mind.

In the *Secret Doctrine of the Goddess Tripura*, a yogini gives this teaching to the proud Astavakra, who claims that nothing in this world is unknown to him:

> "As long as the movement of the intelligence toward the outside has not been suspended, there is no possible inner gaze. As long as there is no inner gaze, one does not attain this pure consciousness. This inner gaze is devoid of all tension or strain: how could it belong to an intellect strained with effort?
>
> "This is why you must approach yourself from your own essence, abandoning any kind of tension or strain. Then, for an instant, you will rejoin your own essence and you will sustain yourself in it without thought. Then you will remember yourself, and you will understand in what sense consciousness is simultaneously both unknowable and perfectly known. Such is the truth. When you have known it, you will reach the immortal state.
>
> "That is all I have to say to you, oh ascetic's son! Now I salute you and am on my way. If you could not understand all this simply by listening, then King Janaka, the best of the sages, will enlighten you. Ask him unceasingly and he will remove all your doubts."

Upon these words, while the king was paying her homage and while all the members of the assembly were bowing down, the yogini disappeared like a cloud chased by the wind.[34]

Easefulness allows immaculate consciousness to emerge; presence in our actions allows this same consciousness to unfold spherically toward the world, to contact it deeply, and to let it come back to the source of the heart, where each perception finds freshness and tremoring vibration.

Thus, as Asanga says in one of the marvelous definitions of what a Bodhisattva is,

> the unceasingly-increasing relaxation and ease of body and Heart allow him [the Bodhisattva] to obtain a fundamental base . . . his body and consciousness having become supple to the highest degree. . . . Having understood that the world is only latent tendencies and being devoid of self and the initial seeds of pain, he eliminates this view of the self which does not aim for the good of others and he takes refuge in the great view of the Self with great benefit because this view is transmitted to the equitable, impartial consciousness of self and other; all beings having been substituted for the "I," this consciousness becomes the source of the disinterested activity of the Bodhisattva in consideration and in the interest and favor of all.[35]

Here, we are far from the idea of the Bodhisattva who refuses to enter nirvana before all people are saved because, for the adherents of Yogacara, the opposing of samsara and nirvana is absent of presence to the world. The state of nirvana infuses all of samsara, and the absolute is found in reality, as Ma-tsu and the Ch'an masters maintain.

A Ch'an story tells of how two adepts, one of the Ch'an school, the other of a different school, meet along a river. The adept of the other school says that his master possesses extraordinary powers. Seated on one side of the river, this master can draw in the air the marks printed on a piece of paper that one of his disciples is holding on the other side of the river. "And your master, of what marvels is he capable?"

"My master is a great magician," answers the Ch'an adept. "When he is thirsty, he drinks; when he is hungry, he eats; when he is tired, he goes to bed."

This is the kind of elegy for simple, ordinary reality that is found all through Ch'an, Yogacara, *dzogchen*, and Kashmiri Shaivism.

Presence becomes more and more firmly established and leads to what the last chapter of the colossal *Avatamsaka Sutra* names "entrance into the kingdom of Reality."

The sage is thus capable of acting with lightning-bolt speed, because dualistic thought no longer paralyzes him. His acts are instantaneous and carriers of light; this is what is called nonaction. The sixth consciousness is short-circuited, the unconscious is no longer buried, and the whole tremoring vibration of the senses constantly comes to celebrate that consciousness from which all movement and action emanate.

# 20

~

# A Question: Freeing Oneself from the Past

Over the course of the seminars I give, I am often asked questions like this:

*I can conceive and realize from actual events that from the moment in which presence to reality is continuous, I can stop storing material in the unconscious, since everything flows into the Self, into immaculate consciousness. But what do I do with the material preceding continuous presence? How do I become free of that? This is a major problem . . .*

The Kashmiri tantrikas resolved this problem, which is indeed a crucial one. For them, there is no succession of time. Only the present exists. Whether we are having a memory of an event or are imagining the future, everything happens in the present. This is what allows the treatment and healing of old wounds, painful emotions.

But there is a specific way to do this. This way is presence to the emotions, to the movements of the body, to the enslavements we suffer under. When the body-mind becomes calm, there are very often jolts of the unconscious, as if it were taking advantage of the clarity of the mind to come to the surface. At this moment, if we succeed, with the suppleness of a tiger, in staying with presence, whatever arises naturally goes toward the sensory. We can then completely feel the first symptoms again and live them without there being any obstruction or any tie to the ego. Then this suffering, rather than returning to the reservoirs of the unconscious, goes directly into immaculate consciousness, meets the source, and is transformed into luminous space.

This is one of the important stages, a kind of massive cleaning of the deepest part of our being. It is a very moving and powerful moment when we feel that all the absorbed marks and refuse of the past are being filtered by absolute consciousness. It is the work of a whole life, a work that comes after awakening, but it is done spontaneously and is not the object of a practice. It cannot be said that when the tiger sets out on the hunt, it is doing its "practice."

When everything that arises is no longer stopped by the mental, ego-tied consciousness, there is then what Asanga and the *Lankavatara Sutra* call "reversal," or "reverse flow"— that is, direct and inalterable flow, toward the heart, into immaculate innermost consciousness. The unconscious is no longer fed, and we recover freedom. This freedom then allows use of the eight consciousnesses, because the tie to the ego no longer happens. Even the discriminating consciousness, the sixth, operates from the deep core of the person, Buddha nature, or Shiva nature within the Self. In this way all that binds, makes suffer, or causes anxiety in the person absent to the world is for the practitioners of Yogacara, Ch'an, and Tantrism the very site of their continuous liberation.

# 21

~

# Scents of the World

When we breathe, we detect the electrical charge of the molecules that enter into contact with the receptors in the nasal cavities. This contact lasts a millisecond, and then our memory restores the smell to us. Starting from our development in the womb, we learn to recognize smells through those of the food that nourishes our mother.

Smells have great importance and are often connected to our tastes. The natural odor of people whom we meet or pass prompts us to immediate reactions of attraction or repulsion, without our being conscious of the origin of these reactions. This sense is very important in our sexual relationships and is a determining factor in our choice of partners, even though our mind provides us with all sorts of "reasons" for our attraction. Women are particularly sensitive to smells, and for all human beings, losing the olfactory sense is accompanied by a loss in sexual interest. Since antiquity perfumes have been an important part of human creativity. They evolve over time, tastes change, but not the attraction that they exert upon us. The craft of the perfume maker is so refined and his apprenticeship so long that it often occurs in a familial setting, because a "nose" is only acquired by starting the apprenticeship at a very tender age. The link between smell and memory is very subtle and is "worked" from the very first years of life, upon entering into contact with all the scents of the world.

Our nose informs us about the food we consume. It also informs some therapists about the mental state of their patients. Anxiety literally has a smell for those gifted with this sensitivity. Some nurses and psychiatrists speak of the particular odor of schizophrenics. Masseuses often smell changes in the body's natural odor when tensions in the body give way to muscular relaxation and pleasure.

The more we lose the natural refinement of this sense, the more the industrialized societies artificially perfume the world. Public places, clothes, cars, airplanes, supermarkets, shopping centers, artificial foods, books, and a good many other things are scented, the aim being to get us to buy.

Our fifty million olfactory cells urge us toward all sorts of pleasures. Sometimes the enchanting allure of a single smell is enough to give us back our taste for life. People who stop smoking experience a whole new emerging universe of smells within a few months of quitting.

The yoga of awareness to our olfactory perceptions allows us entry into an infinite world. Awareness to the smells of things rapidly gives the impression of coming alive again, of regaining the use of a sense that has ensured our survival and has over time become a little unnatural. We will be surprised by all the information our nose provides us, once we allow our consciousness to enter into this activity.

*As soon as I awaken, I become present to the sense of smell. What comes to me as I cross my apartment? The smell of the parquet? The smell of a bouquet of flowers? Of fabric warmed by the sun? Of butter and bread, or the tea or coffee that I prepare? Of the fruit in a bowl? Of a cat that approaches me? Of a child? Of a man or woman?*

*What do the smells of those I meet, those I talk to, those I work with, tell me?*

*When I meditate, the sense of smell can allow me to float far, far away, to open up space infinitely.*

## 22

# Tuning the Body-Instrument to Absolute Love

*T*antrism believes that the body is the temple and that seated at the heart of this temple is divinity. In their teachings the masters of this tradition often refer to the body as a stringed instrument, the *sarangi*, and compare presence to the world with the tuning of this instrument. If a perfectly tuned instrument is left in a room, merely playing another instrument in the same room will set the strings of the first to vibrating. In the same way, we can enter into resonance with the world once we have tuned ourselves. What the tantrikas call yoga is this same work, this game of being perpetually in tune, ready to vibrate to reality such as it unfolds. Doing an experiment of trying to be present to our sensorality for just three minutes is enough to make us realize that a great number of obstacles get us off track from our objective:

- Distraction due to the automatic activity of thought
- Projections
- References to the past
- The discrepancy between what we desire and what we are living

- The contradictions existing between our life and our beliefs
- The feelings of our original sin and our unworthiness
- The desire to modify the tenor of reality
- The desire to be present only to pleasure and to obscure all suffering, tension, anxiety, and unease
- The desire to modify the duration of some elements of reality

Our difficulty in being present comes principally from the fact that we do not accept reality as it is because we see neither its beauty nor its depth. We wrongly imagine that life as we reorchestrate it is more worthy of being lived. Hence we lose considerable energy wanting to transform reality so that it corresponds to our plans, ideals, and beliefs. Unfortunately, reality is not made to conform itself to our desires. Thus do we lose a lot of time in this absurd occupation. That is the chief difficulty in living a more freely flowing, fluid life, one in which reality is no longer frozen by the mind.

The mind is used to, and marvelously capable of, moving quickly and harmonizing with the flow of life, which itself also has great mobility. Every time we intervene to make something that is transitory by nature last, we block the natural flow of life. Every time we intervene in an attempt to cut off a sensation or an emotion that does not correspond to our desires, we paralyze, we block the natural flow of life.

Let's take an example: We meet someone whom we are attracted to. From the first moments, our mind will set itself in motion, get itself going, and we will form a strategy, a plan, expectations, hopes. Fears will immediately come into play. The fear of being wronged or deceived, of being abandoned, will surge up very quickly. We have not yet had the time to develop any real intimacy with this person and yet already our whole system has been put in a position of overabundance and failure. The whole energetic arena of the encounter is already a minefield of strategies, which are all the more disconcertingly surprising and distracting because there are two of us elaborating them. It can be said that this whole conceptual structure will minimize our chances of a true meeting, of a true connection.

Corporality, being present to another, is henceforth jumbled up with an infinite number of encumbrances. Future actions will thus lack spontaneity and intensity—as if we are being tele-guided by distant beings. We will find ourselves once again in this situation in which two people lacking in completeness will, by a sort of mutual cannibalism, attempt to fill the void in their lives. Each will use the other from this perspective and, even if we pass through happy moments, the time will come where the sum of these strategies and blockages will completely paralyze the relationship.

Sentimental and psychological projections, reference to memories, insistence on finally finding what we want—all this will create significant areas of darkness or shadow wherein the story we are in the process of building will get bogged down. Neither grace nor spontaneity will dwell in any part of the unfolding that the extraordinary adventure of a meeting between two people can be. Novelty alone gives us the illusion that this time, at last, we have found our soul mate.

And we hold the same attitude toward objects. If we lose the enthusiasm and incandescence of adolescence, it is not because this loss is inevitable; it is because we fall into the formidable trap of absence to reality.

If we could, however, meet another—if we could come into contact with the world and objects and people—while remaining totally present, we would have an experience of immense freshness. The moment would be full of the total trust that we have in our corporality, in anything felt or sensed, disencumbered of all mental jumble and sentimental projection. At this moment we would be able to live love.

Many people confuse sentimental projection with love. We think they are the same thing. We imagine that a sexual relationship without sentimental projection is something cold and mechanical. Yoginis and yogis believe instead that there can be no profound meeting with another, and hence no love, as long as this sentimental tie exists. Why? Simply because when we use these mental ruses—which is what sentimental projections are—we are not sincere with ourselves. We deceive ourselves just as we deceive the other person. We have a plan for ourselves and for the other person. If she does not conform to this plan, we will be disappointed and resent her for it. Because of this, we are not in tune with ourselves, and we do not give the other person the space for freedom that is indispensable if love is to become manifest.

All our projections, all our expectations, all our desires, all our blockages of the flow of life are thus negations of love's freedom. Love without freedom does not exist. Freedom cannot coexist with the ego, and the ego can only be dissipated by total presence to reality, presence deprived of all fear, all strategy, all planning. Then the only thing remaining is the fundamental desire to be in space, to be in the nonperson, in the nonrelationship—because we are in total and nondual presence.

The only love that can satisfy us is the love that can arise from within us when all projections cease. At this moment no one can cut us off from the source of consciousness. It is precisely presence to the flow of this source that leads to the autonomy yoginis and yogis live. No longer conditioned by ties, they are love and, when they are love, they desire nothing more because they are completely gratified and completely gratify those whose paths they cross.

# 23

## Questions: Love, Sexuality, Fidelity

*How do I reconcile this sphere of spontaneity—which really speaks to me and appeals to me—with the life of a woman who lives in society, has a relationship, wants children; who out of necessity must have plans and carry them out; who feels happy with a man she loves; and for whom fidelity is important? Can I live this sphere of immense openness you talk about and be a "normal" woman, so to speak? How does a Tantric master or an aspiring tantrika live? How do I live out the sexual desire that I can feel for other women and men?*

This is a very interesting question, because it troubles a lot of people. We often think—and I admit that I was the first to do so—this path is too absolute to be lived in the usual social setting. I thought that in order to realize his practice, a tantrika had to live alone, to be completely available. As Abhinavagupta says, "In Tantrism, nothing is advised, nothing is forbidden." The ideal of the Tantric masters is precisely to blend themselves into society, not to be obvious. No marks, no disguises, no isolation. Most Kashmiri masters are married and lead family lives. This is their usual situation and is also the meaning of the word *Kula*, the name of a school of Kashmiri Shaivism. *Kula* means "Tantric family." Yoginis and yogis live in a more isolated way, as was the case with my master Devi, who taught only one person at a time. The personal relationship is so important to the Kashmiri masters that they do not even have ashrams. They teach in the familial setting. Disciples live in the master's and her family's house, and the family takes them under their wing. Sometimes disciples live next door in a village house. Tantrikas are women and men who fill a role in society. They work, they plan, they meet their objectives. Their quest is completely inner. No one suspects they are tantrikas. They are indistinguishable from anyone else. The masters follow the same line of conduct. There are some great Tantric masters who are known by only a few people, so discreet are their lives. One of them spent his life as a beggar in front of the central post office in Bombay. That was his role. At night he received a few disciples. Nisargadatha Maharaj sold "beedies"—little Indian cigarettes made from rolled eucalyptus leaves—and taught while serving his customers, who sometimes became his disciples. It is interesting to see that, often, yoginis and yogis live with a partner. We have many examples of historic masters who followed the teachings of a yogini. They lived and practiced together, sometimes for their whole life, like Naropa and Nigouma, or like Saraha with the arrow-making yogini. Abhinavagupta, in the first stanza of the *Tantraloka*, pays homage to the family:

> Immortal family, unequaled, made from the lightning-flash emission of a couple's union, formed by the father whose body is plenitude and whose five faces house all the splendor, and by the mother whose radiance, in ever-

renewing emissions, is founded on the pure creative power
of energy, how completely my heart blazes!

A little farther on, he pays homage to one of his numerous
masters: "Glory to Sambhunatha, unique being, accompanied by his beloved. . . ." A few stanzas later:

Abhinavagupta teaches this doctrine, he who is made to
blaze with the veneration . . . that he gives to the successive masters and to start at Bhattanatha's lotus feet and
those of the Bhattarika, the venerable lady, his partner.[36]

In the texts, perfected Shaktis who share their life with another master are not passed over in silence.

It should be understood that to live as a tantrika has nothing to do with a rejection of society or a rejection of the ties
that exist between men and women. Everything happens at
a more subtle, refined level. Obviously, life in society does
not happen without planning and without meeting necessary objectives. What Tantric "work" will lead you to discover is a growing intimacy with what you are in reality,
how the society of cells and organs is organized within you,
how this society is animated by movements and actions, by
corporality, by thoughts, desires, and emotions.

Remember, all we do is observe and understand what is.
Therefore, if you have a family life, you observe yourself and
understand yourself in this setting. If you live alone, you gain
an intimacy with that setting. The spontaneity that will slowly
make its home in you will lead you to discover life as it is.
From your own reality everything will unfold, spreading
spherically around you. Presence will change your relationships with those you are close to, as well as those you work
with. How much more you listen to others will increase in
proportion to how much more you listen to yourself.

Presence generates harmony, which is what a family needs. By being present, you will offer freedom to those you are close to as well as to yourself. When we talk about naked awareness, void of intentionality, this does not mean we make no plans; it means we let things establish themselves in their true space, without diverting them by intentionality, which closes off both ourselves and other people. We are present and, in this presence, we allow others to live out their own fundamental freedom to be present themselves. To live as a couple in this way is a never-ending and marvelous practice.

Fidelity, which worries many people, is not a problem. The more fully you live, the more desire will find itself in constant tremoring vibration, with or without an object. This tremoring will come from you, from your consciousness, from your heart, and will shower down both on those close to you and on those you meet. Even those sitting near you on the bus will benefit from it.

And as you drink more and more from your own fountain-source, dissatisfaction will cease to exist, as will outer demands, because it is the whole of life that brings you this loving tremoring. There is no longer something missing to make up for; it is the unrestrained intensity of your desire that fulfills you now, and no longer the ideas of possessing, of seducing, of filling a void, of feeding your dissatisfaction.

Curiously, you will see that the more incandescent your desire, the less it will turn toward objects of desire, because it no longer needs them to mask incompletion. This is what the tantrikas experience and know, and this is what is so misunderstood by those who see Tantrism as a quest for ego-tied sexual satisfaction.

The fact of becoming free by finding completeness will enable you to have unusual relationships with other people—that is to say, truly warm and sensual relationships that involve the whole body-mind and that escape all classification. These relationships will lead you to discover that with each true look, with each profound contact of your relaxed and easeful body, you will receive and transmit the teaching: a peaceful, sensually nourishing, authentic human presence.

Your desire will therefore pour out in a new, continuous way. There will no longer exist an accumulation of energy that can find calm only in orgasmic release. You will enter into a sphere in which you will be unceasingly in the process of making love, and enjoying immense pleasure, coming, with the whole world—which leaves hardly any room for what we call "affairs." You will live the Great Affair, the one that never ends. *That* is the life of an aspirant, of a tantrika, of a yogini, of a master.

# 24

## Chants of the Dakinis, the Great Secret

The *dakini* Nigouma, companion and master of Naropa, sings, in her poem on Mahamudra, the Great Seal, ultimate initiation not only of Tibetan Buddhism of the Kagyu school but also of the Kashmiri schools, that Mahamudra describes the state of supreme and natural awakening of the mind, very close to the *dzogchen*, or Great Perfection:

> *Don't do anything whatsoever with the mind—*
> *Abide in an authentic, natural state.*
> *One's own mind, unwavering, is reality.*
> *The key is to meditate like this without wavering;*
> *Experience the great [reality] beyond extremes. . . .*
>
> *In a pellucid ocean,*
> *Bubbles arise and dissolve again.*
> *Just so, thoughts are no different from ultimate reality,*
> *So don't find fault; remain at ease.*
> *Whatever arises, whatever occurs,*
> *Don't grasp—release it on the spot.*

*Appearances, sounds, and objects are one's own mind;*
*There's nothing except mind.*
*Mind is beyond the extremes of birth and death.*
*The nature of mind, awareness,*
*Although using the objects of the five senses,*
*Does not wander from reality.*

*In the state of cosmic equilibrium*
*There is nothing to abandon or practice,*
*No meditation or post-meditation period.*[37]

To encounter such a being who wants nothing from you, who refuses nothing, who takes nothing, and who does not even want to lead you to liberation is the experience of all those who approach an authentic master. Such frequent contact makes us keen to attain the fluidity that we perceived in the mirror held out to us. A master is nothing else but the mirror of our own freedom. In the total easing and opening of the mind, he has no projections; he allows the richness of each moment to pass before him like a parade and contacts his sensorality without making any mental commentary about it. He lives things as they are, in their intensity and their original duration, without adding, without cutting off, without grasping or abandoning. A master is always there, ready for unconditional love.

The "Corpse-Raising *Dakini*" sings:

*Don't become distracted, but don't meditate;*
*To practice like this is skillfulness.*
*When myriad experiences leave no trace, how great!*
*To practice like this is liberation.*
*KYE HO! Wonderful!*
*Great fresh awareness is the supreme path.*

*No need to walk—it's the ground of suchness.**
*No need to practice, it's effortlessly accomplished.*
*AHA! Those who practice this yoga are fortunate indeed!*[39]

How can someone who longs simply to be an entirely unique human, by using the whole range of her corporality, mind, and emotions, come close to this?

In attempting as often as possible to be present to reality, we will make contact with this reality at certain times, miss it at others. Little by little we will taste things in the depth of presence and in the silence of the mind. From living in this space of freedom a few seconds here, a few seconds there, our whole body-mind will turn more and more spontaneously toward presence, simply because it will discover that nothing brings it deeper satisfaction or deeper pleasure.

As we start to get a taste of reality, we will discover that our presence extends to the whole of our mental and physiological functionings. We will be more and more sensitive to the incredible mass of encumbrances to naked reality that we generate. It is then that our attitude will spontaneously and gently change.

Through consciousness, we discover the ways in which we short-circuit life. Consequently, we never adopt a new way of being or pursue a new ideal, because this would be to enclose ourselves once again in concepts. We observe without judgment, and it is this clarity that will shine light on our behavior and lead us, most naturally, to stop blocking the course of life. In order to liberate ourselves, we will observe that we block and how we block.

Someone who desires to be fully alive has to do nothing

---

*Suchness* might be defined as "the true nature of things, outside of subjective description and all interpretation of what we perceive."[38]

but observe without inner commentary the automatic mechanisms that stop him from tasting the tremoring vibration of life. This observation alone is the key to our liberation. It requires naked and silent awareness, detached from all objectives. A light and fluid, playful and feline attention, with the absolute ease that precedes the movements of the big cats. Yoginis and yogis are often compared to tigresses and tigers, whose skins they sometimes use for meditating, because they have the same intense liveliness, the same vivaciousness.

Little by little we will see that this play totally changes our relationship with others. We will finally be here, without expectation or plan, without fear, without the need to grasp or reject. We will then feel a profound peace distilled all through our sensitive body, which will have become complete presence and tremoring vibration to the other. The two instruments will be able to tune themselves to each other and vibrate in unison.

In the absence of mental commentary, our entire sensorality will be able to come into a state of vibration and pick up the vibration of the other. In this silence nothing is planned, nothing whose real duration we have not accepted. Nothing that we attempt to increase or make last. Simply movement, flow, plenitude in their intrinsic reality, which nothing comes along to strain or reduce. The spontaneous dawning of acts, deeds, movements, gestures will then make contact with an unknown grace, with a magic all the more real because it is moving and free.

When we have tasted this kind of communication, we will understand to what extent this connection reveals the fundamental freedom of all people, and we will naturally tend toward letting it overflow into all our relationships, simply because we will have lived, in these moments of ecstasy, the experience of being both people and objects. At this point there will no longer be relation to other, which is what the tantrikas call presence to reality.

This is also what Bhaskara tells us in his commentary on the *Shiva Sutras:* "The senses have the power to make this new creation emerge, as experience proves, because they are sustained by the inborn power of consciousness. It is thus because the power of the senses comes from the absorbing force existing in the Self."

# 25

## Looking at the World

The functioning of the sense of sight is extremely complex and occupies an important part of our brain. The eye is a marvel of sophistication. The molecules of our retina respond to tremorings of light and our brain replicates the visible world by restoring to it color, movement, perspective, depth of field, texture, and form.

Sight functions even when we have our eyes closed. Dreams and the imagination allow us to see what the eye is not physically seeing. Memory restores striking images to us. Yogis and yoginis use visualization to practice the yoga of lineage or the yoga of different divinities into which they transform themselves over the course of different *sadhanas*.

The Tibetans have carried the art of visualization to a level of extraordinary refinement. Through visualization, yogis and yoginis create imaginary worlds in the forms of mandalas, which they bring forth from vacuity and into which they reimmerse themselves after having identified themselves with the divinity. The symbolic universe is hence created and dissolved in the infinite space of vacuity.

In Kashmiri Shaivism visualizations are more rarely used, and awareness is wholly and entirely turned toward full consciousness of what our sight perceives. Aesthetic emotion is considered a place of ideal tremoring vibration where the whole, reunified person completes the endless circle that rises from consciousness in a continual flow, caresses the world, and leads this acute intensity back to consciousness in a constant movement.

The *Vijnanabhairava Tantra* enumerates a number of practices concerning the sense of sight. One of the favorite occupations of yoginis and yogis consists of watching the sky, which has a mindlike nature, until the moment wherein union with space takes place. I spent nights shivering, lying on the freezing ground, my body completely abandoned, often at the end of an outlandish race through the woods with Devi. This meditation can be practiced at dawn, at twilight, or in the middle of the night. Abandoned to the stars.

It is said that Bodhidharma, after his confrontation with the Emperor of the Weis, spent nine years contemplating a wall at the Shao-lin monastery. Even today practitioners of Ch'an and certain Zen schools meditate with their eyes open in front of a wall. This is an excellent practice that empties the mind of all forms.

---

*I become conscious of the involuntary movements of my eyes and eyelids. I see how I interrupt communication by incessant blinking. Looking into space, without focusing on any particular point, I learn to communicate, to be the other, to be the object of my contemplation. I rediscover the peaceful gaze of the child who studies the world. I rediscover the peace of the gaze that wants nothing.*

*Little by little, I transform each blink into a conscious act. I become conscious of the way in which the eye naturally moistens itself. I note the difference in communication that is established when I truly look at people and things.*

*I let my gaze find rest by taking the time to require nothing of it. I allow my gaze to go out and meet the world by avoiding the hyperactivity that masks my reality. I caress textures. I allow my gaze to be the mirror of consciousness.*

# 26

## Passion

Passion is, for the Tantric masters of the various traditions, an element indispensable to the spiritual search and the plenitude of life. For them, everything is movement, emission and retraction, enjoyment, creativity, incandescence. Even to give themselves over to meditation, they believe a certain degree of excitation *(harsa)* is necessary. Swami Lakshmanjoo writes: "Unless you fall in love with meditation and approach it with total enthusiasm, attachment, and longing, you cannot enter the realm of Awareness."[40]

It could be said that the Tantric masters have a very simple approach to life and that we can follow their advice without having to adhere to any ideal other than to become a unique human being, using the whole range of these capacities in order to come deeply into contact with life. In certain paths initiation to this simplicity is preceded by a long and tedious training; the supreme truth is revealed only to those who have successfully passed through years of *sadhana*.

In Kashmiri Shaivism as taught by my master, Lalita Devi, this truth about the real nature of the mind is taught immediately, and the means by which it can be completely realized are put into play right from the start of the relationship. But my Tibetan master, Kalou Rinpoche, introduced me to the real nature of the mind—Mahamudra, the Great Seal—only after my work with Devi. He wrote in *Luminous Mind: The Way of the Buddha:* "When transformation of the emotions [Mahamudra] is fully completed, the passions are no longer an obstacle. They even become a help. A traditional image is that they become like wood for the bonfire of wisdom; the more you add, the brighter the flame!"[41]

Earlier, he says:

In itself, the practice of Mahamudra is extremely simple and easy. There are no visualizations or complicated exercises. There is nothing *to do*. It is enough just to leave the mind in its natural state, *as it is, as it comes, without contrivance*. It is extremely simple. In the tradition of mahamudra reliquary,* it is said that mahamudra is:

- Too close to be recognized,
- Too deep to grasp,
- Too easy to believe,
- Too amazing to be understood intellectually.

Those are the four obstacles that prevent its recognition.[42]

One day I was surprised to see a Kashmiri master refuse to take on a disciple who seemed to be a very serious practitioner. When I asked him the reason for this refusal, he told me: "Not passionate enough. I do not see the quality of tremoring vibration that we like to work with."

An impassioned person—even if this passion is manifested in hardly orthodox ways, by outrageous exuberance,

---

*Kalou Rinpoche's note: See the Five Golden Teachings in the Vajrayana (213).

a difficult personality, outbursts of violent feelings, actions deemed inappropriate—will have every chance of pleasing a Tantric master, on the condition that behind all of it is true generosity.

The case of Lalla, the poet and Kashmiri master of the fourteenth century, is typical. From the age of twelve, Lalla had mystical experiences. She performed miracles, one of which was to elude the fury of her husband, who was attempting to bludgeon her skull with a club. He only succeeded, however, in breaking the earthenware jar she was carrying on her head, while the water retained the shape of the jar.

Lalla, exuberant, convinced her guru, the Siddha Shrikantha, to give her the teachings by defecating on an image of Shiva that was in the guru's house. When Shrikantha asked her the reason for this act, Lalla replied: "If Shiva is everywhere, he is also in the dirt of the dumping grounds where I usually go. If every place is sacred, why bother choosing?" Convinced by this young aspirant, Shrikantha agreed to give her the teachings after a long wait. Lalla exults over this event in one of her poems:

> *At last the guru gave me the teachings.*
> *He told me: "Stop turning your attention toward the outside;*
> *Fix it on the Self instead."*
> *I carried this truth in my Heart*
> *And then I started dancing, naked!*

Later, Lalla experienced the awakening of the kundalini:

> *When differentiating mind is lulled and sleeps,*
> *The Kundalini awakens!*
> *The five senses' source gushes forth forever.*
> *The water of unceasing presence to the world*
> *Is sweet, and I offer it to Shiva.*

*The unending sacred tremoring of consciousness*
*Is the supreme state.*[43]

This marvelous incandescence, this passion, is the particular mark of all the tantrikas. In order to find it, the adept must seize things in their very first tremorings, before differentiating thought intervenes. It is at this instant that the difference is made between a hedonist, whose worldly search is tied to the ego, and the tantrika, who is in search of the most profound spontaneity.

## 27

Questions: Passion, Ego, Freedom

*How do I recognize the difference between real passion—an act of the senses that unfolds from a yoga point of view, spherically as you say—and one that is simply coming from an ego-tied search for pleasure?*

When the ego enters into play, this is accompanied by a mental performance. We anticipate, we judge, we weigh the forthcoming pleasure by trying to know in what way this pleasure will truly satisfy us. We become strained and tense. Our mind becomes agitated. We set up a choice, we apply a strategy, we grasp onto the object of our desire, use it, and then reject it once we are satisfied. We do this with people, with objects, with our senses, emotions, and our thoughts. We feed ourselves like predators. We impoverish the world in our own interest, we cause harm, we reveal that an unhealthy love is at work.

What does a tantrika do? When a stimulation arises, it is only the expression of the tantrika's own inner tremoring vibration. She relaxes, gets herself in tune, opens her sensitivity, allows the source of the heart to emerge freely. Through her movements and actions, plenitude expresses itself. Her mind remains peaceful, without waves. In each impassioned tremoring vibration, she recognizes the tremoring vibration of her own consciousness. She tastes the world without destroying its harmony. She does not grasp; she does not accumulate. A thing or a person comes up: She meets it with naked presence. This person or thing disappears: She stays in the flow of presence, aware of the entirely new splendor of what just appeared to her. Nothing is fixed; she gets hooked by, hooks onto, nothing. Her life perpetually renews itself, and her peaceful mind does not hinder the course of things. She keeps herself in the natural state of the mind that her master revealed to her. Stable, steady, tremoring to her inner vibration, sensitive, and present, she plays, intention-free, to the rhythm of reality and in this way, each moment, she realizes her true nature.

*But is this not an egoist attitude? Where is compassion in this approach?*

We cannot do a greater good to another human being than to accord him our naked awareness, devoid of all plan. This is the very space of freedom, which he will get a taste of through our presence. In this respect for the other, a mirror without any smudges of volition is presented. The other person can hence see his own freedom and see that there is no longer any separation from the world. *That* is love. Tantrikas hardly ever use the word *compassion*, because it implies a slightly condescending duality, whereas love is a non-differentiated state.

A person who feels loved in such a way feels liberated from mental elaboration and finds herself plunged into the deepest practice of yoga. If she succeeds in getting a taste of this state, the nostalgia for unity comes back to her and, naturally, she will glide toward a more and more silent, a deeper and deeper presence to the world. What more can one give to a human being?

*But the ideal of the Bodhisattva, in Buddhism, isn't it exactly to refuse to enter into nirvana as long as all human beings have not reached it?*

The Bodhisattva does not differentiate between nirvana and samsara. For him, full consciousness of reality is nirvana. He therefore has no place to go to and even less to wait for, because there is no duality between worldly experience and nirvana. There also is no difference between the Bodhisattva and the person whom a Bodhisattva could help. It is this nondifferentiation between the states of nirvana and samsara, this nondifferentiation between people, this nondifferentiation between subject and object that liberates people. Everything, for the Bodhisattva, happens in the consciousness of an absolute nature. "The fact that this consciousness is neither associated, nor non-associated with attraction, aversion, confusion, or hindrances—here is the pure luminosity of consciousness," reads one sutra.

*Can it be said, then, that it is all right for a practitioner to experiment with pleasure? Certain masters say that desire and passions must be cut off to attain awakening.*

If you think desire and passions must be cut off, do it. Put all your energy into this project and see after a while if the flames of desire and passions have gone out in you. Examine the situation clearly. Have you found plenitude? Are you emancipated from desires and passions? Take a little tour around the city; come out of your retreat. Walk around; watch people. Are you really emancipated from desires and passions? Then examine the state of your sensitivity of perception. Has it developed, or on the contrary has it become weakened, wilted, withered? Do certain expressions of the body, voices, emotions, desires of others bother you? Have you found a joyous stability, an enthusiasm in the face of life? Is there no coldness or hardness in your gaze, in your body, in your mind? If this is the case, if nothing disturbs you anymore, you have succeeded.

This is an extremely difficult undertaking. Man-An, the seventeenth-century Zen master, has said, drawing on a stanza from the poem by the Third Patriarch of Ch'an, Seng t'san:

The Third Patriarch of Zen said, "If you want to head for the Way of Unity, do not be averse to the objects of the six senses [the mind is the sixth sense]." This does not mean that you should indulge in the objects of the six senses; it means that you should keep right mindfulness continuous, neither grasping nor rejecting the objects of the six senses in the course of everyday life, like a duck going to water without its feathers getting wet.

If, in contrast, you despise the objects of the six senses and try to avoid them, you fall into escapist tendencies and never fulfill the Way of Buddhahood. If you clearly see the essence, then the objects of the six senses are themselves meditation, sensual desires are themselves the Way of Unity, and all things are manifestations of Reality. Entering into the great Zen stability undivided by movement and stillness, body and mind are both freed and eased.

As for people who set out to cultivate spiritual practice with aversion to the objects and desires of the senses, even if their minds and thoughts are empty and still and their contemplative visualization is perfectly clear, still when they leave quietude and get into active situations, they are like fish out of water, like monkeys out of trees.[44]

But integrating the whole of the desires and the passions with the quest is also a difficult path, because this path demands total clarity about what you really are, with no reference to what you would like to be. By this patient examination you will come to know and discover yourself in reality. You will bring to the light of day all your psychological functionings, your whole sensorality, your thoughts, and your feelings.

Rather than straining toward an objective such as liberating yourself from desire, which is a desire itself, you will enter a virgin space where the fundamental freedom of your consciousness will surface little by little. By slipping into the flow of life, you will have the joyous and luminous experience that the Tantric masters talk about. You will at last be present to reality, not to your objectives, and in this shadowless, maskless reality you will little by little discover the infinite. At this point, you will no longer be anything but love and source. "Everything that flows is good," I once heard someone say.

# 28

## Entrance into the Kingdom of Reality, Cosmic Sensuality

"The five objects of the senses constitute the expanded Cosmos. Of all this knowledge is the Essence. Yoga is liberation," we read in the Kaula Upanishad.[45] This absolute approach of the senses, the emotions, the mind, and the body, which regain their friendly balance in this form of yoga—which in turn involves being deeply involved in our life and surpassing our blockages and our limits—is a larger, all-encompassing approach to existence. The slightest ego-related impulse transforms this subtle, refined, and divine palette into ties with which we will continue to struggle unsuccessfully.

Abhinavagupta, in his commentary on the *Paratrisika*, offers a very profound vision of what the Tantric masters consider liberation lived through the opening of the senses and of sexuality:[46]

Now whatever enters the psychic apparatus of the outer senses of all beings, that abides as sentient life-energy *(cetanarupenaa pranatmana)* in the middle channel i.e., *susumna* whose main characteristic is to enliven all the parts of the body. That life energy is said to be *"ojas"* (vital luster), that is then diffused as an enlivening factor in the form of common seminal energy *(virya)* in all parts of the body.\* Then when an exciting visual or auditory perception enters the recipient, then on account of its exciting power, it fans the flame of passion in the form of the agitation of seminal energy. . . .\*\* Every kind of plea-sure, in a sense, every emotion is conceived as a distur-bance of this force (Raniero Gnoli).

Of the form, sound, etc., even a single one, because of its being made powerful by the augmented vigour re-ferred to previously, can bring about the excitement of the senses pertaining to all other objects also. Since ev-erything is an epitome of all things for all people, even memory or idea of a thing can surely bring about agita-tion because of the excitement of innumerable kinds of experiences like sound etc. lying subconsciously in the omnifarious mind. Only well-developed seminal energy *(virya)* containing the quintessence of all experiences *(paripusta-sarvamaya-mahaviryameva)* can bring about full development and endow one with the power of procre-ation *(pusti-srstikari)*, not its immature state *(apurnam)* as is the case of a child, or its diminished state *(ksinam)* as in the case of an old man. When the seminal energy that has been lying within and identical with one's Self in a

---

\* This means that it contains the *ojas* or vital luster of *sabda* (sound), *rupa* (form), *rasa* (savor), *gandha* (smell), *sparisa* (touch).

\*\* "This 'force,' or rather consciousness itself, is conceived as a kind of emission which incessantly renews the world. Such an emission of force (this force is identified in turn as seed) is the effect of the union of two opposing principles, Shiva and [Feminine, Shakti] Power, Sun and Moon, etc." (Raniero Gnoli).

"Inundated by the beautified emission which issues from the union of the genital organs of Shiva and the Power [Shakti], all this is renewed incessantly" (TA, V, 124).

placid state *(svamayatvena abhinnasyapi)* is agitated *(viksobha)* i.e. when it is in an active state, then the source of its pleasure is the Supreme I-Consciousness full of creative pulsation, beyond the range of space and time *(adesakalakalitaspandamayamahavima-rsa-rupameva)*, of the nature of perfect Bhairava-consciousness, the absolute sovereignty, full of the power of bliss.

Even a (beautiful) figure brought into prominence by the meeting of two eyes affords delight only by the device of its union* with the mighty seminal energy *(mahavisarga-vislesan**-yuktya)* which stirs up the energy of the eyes *(tadviryaksobhatmaka);* such is also the case when the ears hear a sweet song.

In the case of other sense-organs also, the perception by itself (i.e., without its union with the seminal energy) cannot acquire full expansion because of the springing up of energy only in the sense organ itself *(svatmani eva ucchalanat).*[†]

So is the case of those in whom the seminal energy has not developed *(tadvirya-anupabrmhitanam)*, in whom

---

* *Vislesana* here means *visesena slesah*, definite junction or unon. *Mahavisarga-vislesana* is a technical word of the system which means that all joy arises by union with the perfect-consciousness.

"The separation of the emission is the equivalent, in a psychological sense, to the seminal emission. Each form of pleasure can be, from this point of view, conceived as a separation of the emission. From a cosmic point of view, the separation of the emission is equivalent in the end to the creation of the all, contained implicitly in consciousness" (Raniero Gnoli).

**Vislesana* in this context means not separation but union: *visesena slesanam* i.e. uniting in a definite characteristic way.

[†] "The two aesthetic senses are, according to Indian thinkers, sight and hearing. Things perceived through the other senses spring up only in the self proper; they are so to speak incapable of breaking the barriers of the limited ego and the practical interests tied to the ego" (Raniero Gnoli).

the pleasure of love that excites the seminal energy as in other cases, is absent, who are like stone, to whom the beautiful figure of a charming young woman with large and handsome hips, with face moving to and fro with sweet, soft and melodious song cannot give full delight. To the extent to which an object cannot bring about full excitement, to that extent it can provide only limited delight. If there is complete absence of delight, it only spells insentiency. Engrossment in a profuse delight alone excites the seminal energy and that alone signifies a taste for beautiful things *(sahrdayata)*. Excessive delight is possible only to those whose heart is expanded by seminal energy which has the boundless capacity to strengthen sensibility and which is established in them by repeated association with objects of enjoyment. . . .

When there is the dissolution of *prana* and *apana (marudadi)*, in *susumna* which, as the central channel, is full of the storage of the energy of all the senses, then one's consciousness gets entry into that stage of the great central *susumna* channel where it acquires union with the pulsation of one's Sakti *(nijasakti-ksobha-tadatmyam)*, then all the sense of duality dissolves, and there is the perfect I-consciousness generated by the abundance of the perfection of one's own inherent Sakti. Then by one's entry into the union of Siva and Sakti *(rudrayamalayoga-nupravesena)* which consists in the bliss of their essential nature of manifestation and by one's complete integration *(vislesana)* with the expansive flow of the energy of the great *mantra* of perfect I-consciousness, there is the manifestation of the *akula* or *anuttara* (absolute) Bhairava-nature which is beyond all differentiation *(nistaranga)*, unalterable and eternal *(dhruvapadatmaka)*.

In the case of both sexes sustained by the buoyancy of their seminal energy, the inwardly felt joy of orgasm (*antahsparsa sukham*) in the central channel induced by the excitement of the seminal energy intent on oozing out at the moment of thrill (*kampakale sakalavirya-ksobhojigamisatmakam*) is a matter of personal experience to everyone. This joy is not simply dependent on the body which is merely a fabricated thing. If at such a moment it serves a token of remembrance of the inherent delight if the Divine Self (*tadabhijnanopadesadvarena*) (i.e. if at such a moment one realizes *khecari-samya*), one's consciousness gets entry in the eternal, unalterable state (*dhruvapade*) that it realizes by means of the harmonious union (*vislesana*) with the expansive energy of the perfect I-consciousness which constitutes the venerable Supreme Divine Sakti (*parabhattarikarupe*) who is an expression of the absolutely free manifestation of the bliss of the union of Siva and Sakti denoting the Supreme Brahman. It will be said later that "one should worship the creative aspect of the perfect I-consciousness" (*Paratrisika*, Verse 29b). . . .

"O goddess, even in the absence of a woman, there is a flood of delight, simply by the intensive recollection of sexual pleasure in the form of kissing [lit. licking], embracing, pressing, etc." (*Vijnana Bhairava*, Verse 70).*

The above has been said in the following sense:

Even when the contact with a woman is intensely remembered, that is reflected in the sexual organ (*tatsparsa-ksetre*)

---

* Author's note: This stanza is translated on the Tantra/Ch'an Web site as: "O goddess! The sensual pleasure of the intimate bliss of union can be reproduced at any moment by the radiant presence of the mind which remembers intensely this pleasure."

and in the central channel pertaining to the natural, supreme Sakti* *(madhyama-akrtrima-paratmaka-saktinalikapratibim-bitah)*. Then even in the absence of contact with an actual woman *(tanmukhyasaktasparsabhave'pi)*, the intensive memory of the contact excites the seminal energy pertaining to contact with women which lies in it (the central channel). In this connection, it has been said, "At the time of sexual intercourse with a woman, complete union with her is brought about by the excitement which terminates in the delight of orgasm. This only betokens the delight of Brahman which in other words is that of one's own self" *(Vijnana Bhairava, Verse 69)*.**

---

* "The middle or central channel, the *susumna*, is consciousness itself" (Raniero Gnoli).

** Author's note: From the Tantra/Ch'an Web site: "At the start of the union, be in the fire of the energy released by the intimate sensual pleasure. Merge in to the divine Shakti and keep burning in space, avoiding the ashes at the end. These delights are in truth those of the self." This pleasure, in other words, can also be reproduced without the actual presence of a woman, quite simply by concentrating on the woman. See also my translation of the *Vijnanabhairava Tantra* in *Tantra Yoga*.

# 29

## The Sexual Ritual, Maithuna, and the Path of the Left Hand

During Tantric gatherings in Kashmir, the adepts who practice the sexual ritual are placed to the left of the master, the others to his right—hence the expressions *path of the left hand* and *path of the right hand*. But because they are seated in a circle, there comes a moment when the left is no longer different from the right. By extension, those who practice the three Ms—that is, consume meat *(mamsa)* occasionally, ingest alcohol or hallucinatory substances *(madya)*, and practice sexual union *(maithuna)*—are considered practitioners of the left hand. But more generally, it can be said that an authentic master practices with the entirety of what is; even without having received the sexual transmission, she can be considered a practitioner of the left hand once intense emotions and feelings are integrated into the path. Even the most gentle master will occasionally be a master of the left hand when the disciple must be made to confront fundamental fear.

When I was face to face with Devi, I had the constant feeling that she was overjoyed with the whole spectrum of human possibilities—and that her initiation called upon both paths, sometimes even within the space of a few seconds. This is the manner in which I strive to transmit the teachings.

Fundamentally, these divisions are the divisions of the puritan academics, who use this duality to condemn the path of the left hand. These divisions do not correspond to reality. Most Tantric masters consider themselves practitioners of the path of the left hand, even those who live in chastity.

The *maithuna* ritual has made a lot of ink flow, and rare are the Westerners who have received initiation into it by an authentic master. As I received it, this initiation—you may come to understand it by reading Abhinavagupta's texts—is one of the tremoring vibration of all the senses, which return through it to their home, consciousness. For us, there is no difference between a sexual, genital relationship and the sensory relationship that we enter into with the reality that is all around us. What the masters call the Great Union sometimes refers to the sexual union, as is the case in stanzas 69, 70, and 71 of the *Vijnanabhairava Tantra,* but often the Great Union refers to the union of the sensory mass with the world, as is stated in the *Vatulanatha Sutra:* "The Great Union proceeds from the unification of the senses with their objects."[47] For the tantrika, activity does not lead to consciousness but proceeds from it and returns to it after having united itself with the object. Nothing comes from the outside.

Consciousness flows like a spring toward the world, comes into deep contact with it, at its incandescent and tremoring core, and returns to consciousness in continuous circulation. *Maithuna* is the recognition that this freedom has already been attained by the aspirant and that the fruits of the yoga are ripe. In absolutely no case is it a ritual in the sense of a magic act that would allow a taste of a state of plenitude lacking in us beforehand.

In order to aspire to initiation, it is necessary to have realized that desire does not know how to, cannot, be satisfied by an object, and that incandescence is what remains when the desire *for something* has been consumed. To celebrate this state of abandon, the master gives (or not) the initiation or the transmission of *maithuna* once the disciple has joined him in completeness. If something is lacking, there is no initiation. Tremoring and continual *samadhi* is the narrow doorway into *maithuna,* because the union symbolizes the prior union of the tantrika with the universe.

Besides, many masters give it through the gaze, a lucid dream, nongenital contact, the voice, or the mind. Sexuality is not the only means of access; it is equal to all other manifestations of sensorality, one site of consciousness. What is more, out of 120 or 130 *Vijnanabhairava Tantra* practices, only 4 concern *maithuna,* which shows to what extent sexuality, in our usual sense of the word, is integrated into the whole.

Practically speaking, there is an abandon to the profound breath, which eliminates any difference between master and disciple; at this point identity is celebrated by the Great Union. Then orgasm no longer needs the release of ejaculation, because the tantrika has integrated feminine energy. Moreover, a woman who is not open to the world is considered energetically a man by the tantrikas. At the energetic level, there is therefore only woman, the presence of Shakti.

The Tantric ideal is that of integration of the male-female duality with plenitude. Shiva is often represented as a hermaphrodite. It is of utmost importance to really understand that consciousness is not unveiled by sudden fits or any use of energetic exercises, agitation, gesticulations, pseudoshamanic dances, and other popular tidbits of "doing" in what is sold in the West under the name of Tantra—but, rather, by the slow and gentle emergence of objectless love, which calmly waits for us to stop pursuing the unattainable.

Seekers, at a deep level, do not long for sexual union with the one they follow but for the unveiling of the Self. Sexual desire for the master, which I experienced intensely, is only one beautiful stage of the abandonment of attachments; this desire must be passed through skillfully without stops along the way, and moving on to the act with a disciple on the path of completeness is the most serious of all the stops. When there are neither taboos nor puritanism, nor thirst for power, nor aspirations to be a master, nor limit, there is no moving on to the act: Everything is only harmony, grace, and spontaneity. Devi allowed me to live this total incandescence, and *that* is the splendor of *maithuna.*

If most authors circle around the question of the "secret" ritual of the Great Union without succeeding in offering a very clear image of it, this is simply because they lack experience and because, without this experience, it is difficult to navigate the jungle of texts, often written in allusive or symbolic language. The Tantras themselves are not always of much help and give rise to multiple interpretations.

In the reality of initiation, once the well-established practices of the yoga of presence, and when the presence of *samadhi*—or "pure presence to reality," as certain Tantric masters define it—are attained, the preparatory work toward sexual initiation can take place. It unfolds in several stages and differs for men and for women.

This fairly long training is based on awareness of the previously unconscious physical processes. It involves penetrating this unknown territory of intense enjoyment, of coming, in a series of subtle, refined methods. From the moment this consciousness finds its home in us during regular sexual relations, particular exercises are implemented in order to arrive at yogic ecstasy.

# 30

*The Tantric Orgasm for Women*

$S$it in a meditation pose and practice slow and gentle breathing, including the movements of the pelvis, leaning backward with the inhalation, completely releasing the belly, leaning forward with the exhale, pulling in the belly. Devi would say that in order to do this movement well, you could imagine yourself as a form of Shakti uniting herself with a perfectly immobile *linga* that she allows to slip into herself by this gentle and continual movement. This breath is essential because it will be implemented, alternately with the partner, during the union ritual.

Become aware of the deep muscles and relax, at the same time, the lower belly, the thighs, and the pubococcygeal muscles, both vaginal and anal. Really relax your spinal column, your neck, your arms and hands, and also your jaw, lips, tongue, eyes.

Lie down, legs apart, and continue to breathe gently in total consciousness of the pelvis, being sensitive to the wavelike movement of the spine all the way down to the coccyx.

Very gently, contract the anus while inhaling for three

seconds. Release it with the exhale three times.

With a slightly stronger contraction, feel the area of muscles expanding using the same breath.

Contract more deeply while lengthening the breath, twelve times. In this way the whole perineum area and the vaginal muscles can be felt.

The perineum is the center of a figure-eight. Above are the vaginal muscles; below, the anal muscles. The contractions, at first, will make the two areas vibrate; then, progressively, you will be able to distinguish the eight muscles of this area.

Progressively, the breath exhaled, hold the contraction for five, ten, fifteen, twenty seconds; then release completely and breathe very gently while moving the pelvis. This contraction will produce a very pleasing warmth, a vibration, a pleasant tremoring, of all the muscles and sometimes of the coccyx. Always follow the contractions with a period of deep relaxation.

Gradually, there will be a differentiation of the vaginal and anal muscles, as well as a deep consciousness of the cervix. This consciousness will lead to the discovery of the vaginal coils, like a series of corresponding rings that little by little contract like a wave descending toward the cervix and rising again, guided by the rhythm of the breath.

Working these muscles requires time and brief but frequent practices. The more relaxed the body at the time of the practice, the more fruitful the practice.

Women have no exercises to do in terms of orgasm, since it is the succession of orgasms that will lead the yogini and yogi to the peak of motionless ecstasy and continuous tremoring vibration.

It is most important to understand that these practices are not done in order to obtain consciousness; instead, consciousness precedes the work.

It sometimes happens that masters initiate women to these practices right at the beginning of the *sadhana* because they are beneficial to the overall functioning and toning of the whole urogenital system. They also have a balancing effect. Starting from the first menstrual cycle, a young woman can therefore put them into practice even if she never takes up sexual yoga.

This work will be accompanied by constant consciousness of the abdominal muscles and of the breath. Continual presence to the breath is the foundation of all the practices of the yoga of presence to reality.

Contrary to what happens in regular sexual relationships wherein excitement mounts with acceleration of the breath, Tantrism teaches us to begin the union by letting ourselves go with this rapid acceleration; then, from the first orgasms, we let ourselves go toward the intensity by progressively slowing down the rhythm of the breath alternating between the two partners.

*31*

~~~

# The Tantric Orgasm
for Men

The work of the Tantric orgasm is the same for men as for women, but it is accompanied by the dissociation of orgasm and ejaculation. In this respect, most authors talk about "controlling the ejaculation." On the contrary, it is really about abandoning all control in a very deep relaxation and easing of the breath.

Many Kashmiri masters, including Devi, use massage as a kind of yoga. Thanks to the contemplative state of the masseur, the person receiving the massage can, little by little, let go totally and allow a marvelous consciousness of the body to emerge, which brings great freshness and spontaneity. That is one of the beauties of this Kashmiri work, where the body is unceasingly kept in tremoring vibration so that consciousness may entirely occupy it. By the massage of points situated on the meridians, the respiratory functions relax. The diaphragm becomes more supple, and the deep muscles release. The whole pelvic region finds an autonomy and an easeful relaxation, both of which will permit progressively and successfully "forgetting about" ejaculation without holding back anything whatsoever. Those who think that tantrikas hold back anything at all have not assimilated the basic principles of total physical and mental relaxation and ease. A mind that produces nothing in the course of a sexual relation, in association with a body that lets go totally: This is the practice of the tantrikas. This practice is of course impossible unless consciousness is profoundly liberated throughout the whole body-mind.

Every man knows that the very idea of holding back engenders physical and mental tension detrimental to the abandon of sexual relations. A man who holds back is in a position of flight compared to the woman, who "gives herself." This attitude establishes a break in communication, a divergence of mind that slips toward a divergence of sensitivity in desire.

If the tantrikas thought about and perfected this feminization of the male reflexes, it is in large part thanks to the teaching of the yoginis supported by all the male masters. Their aim is to open us to the ecstatic duration, to the continuous tremoring garnered by the open senses of the yoginis and yogis. Ecstasy is for them a natural state. All our energetic reflexes block this flow, particularly ejaculation. In order for a man to be able to follow a woman on the successive waves of pleasure, he has but one solution: to become a woman energetically. That is, to abandon himself totally, let go, surrender, completely.

When sexual excitement no longer finds its usual relationship with the ego, it is space that penetrates the man and the woman. They are said then to be "clothed in space," or "dancing in the infinite sky," not only to indicate that they love, like Lalla, to go around naked, but also to mean that they are innerly naked and have become space.

The massage of points situated around the pubis allows us, once the respiratory points have been liberated at the diaphragmatic and abdominal levels, to attain an uninhibited breath, whose depth and slowness will permit the miracle of orgasm without ejaculation.

Contrary to the usual ways, the sexual rhythm of yogis starts in impassioned ardor, where everything works toward bringing excitement to its peak. The more the union is prolonged, the more the rhythm will slow down, until the point of total immobility. All the processes will tend toward calmness while ecstasy itself will follow a lightninglike mounting.

From a practical point of view, the yogini who has taken on the mission of training a tantrika for the Great Union will test his progress on the path of abandon by using all kinds of ways to stimulate him sexually. Those who practice holding back are then demasked. No holding back can resist the skillful stimulating of a sensual woman or a Shakti.

When ejaculation happens, it is not a failure: The yogini will use it to help the aspirant become conscious of the ejaculatory process with its very rapid succession of phases. Sometimes, in the beginning, the yogini will use the various pressure points *(banda)* at the perineum level or two fingers above the right breast, which are designed to short-circuit ejaculation. But these are only temporary tricks to prove to the aspirant that he can let himself go all the way to orgasm without any plan of holding back and that, despite this, ejaculation will not take place. This is, at first, a veritable revelation for a man.[48]

Little by little the habit of relaxing mentally and physically in relation to a goal will become established. The aspirant will totally relax the breath and, one day, the dexterous yogini will no longer press one of the inhibitory points; then, in total surprise, the aspirant will experience one, then a rapid succession of orgasms without ejaculating. If women often need, in order to go from one orgasm to the next, a period of time to rebuild excitement, they will discover that with total relaxation this time of building up energy again is no longer necessary. Each partner can thus cross the different stages of excitement until subtle levels are reached, where orgasm will be quasi-continual or in any case very long, for both.

Through the course of the night, placed in the center of the magic diagram *(yantra)*, where each is recognized as an incarnation of the divine, Shakti-Shiva, by ritual touching of all parts of the body *(nyasa)*, yogini and yogi will reach the state of immobility, without any voluntary contraction but in a total abandon to the tremoring vibration in a union that lasts a whole night. When the initiator is an authentic master, this experience can open into a rising of the kundalini—in other words, to the presence of Shakti in the form of energy. Because in our school the kundalini is liberated through the opening of the heart and not by the working of the lower centers, it is a gentler, more spherical experience than those described by the various authors who have had the experience or who describe those of others.[49]

# 32

## The Group
## Sexual Ritual

The group ritual, even more than the individual ritual, has been the object of all kinds of attacks. Puritan academics, as well as members of other spiritual movements, have wanted to believe that the group ritual involved a symbolic language or a "depraved" practice of the Tantrism of the path of the left hand led by certain small offshoot groups of sectarians. In order truly to understand the spirit of this ritual, it is indispensable to be familiar with what Abhinavagupta, supreme authority of Kashmiri Shaivism, says about it in his *Tantraloka*. We will see that he places this experience first and foremost from the point of view of the body glorified by the yoga of presence, a body made sensitive and tremoring by the yoga of the senses.

Considered the supreme vehicle of divinity, this body is devoid of ego. Having passed beyond desire and object of desire, it can experience the Great Union, which is performed like a sacred ritual wherein all the participants of the spiritual family (Kula) are united through the master with Shiva-Shakti in nondifferentiation. Abhinavagupta furthermore places himself among the practitioners of the path of the left hand in his *Tantrasara* when he speaks of the nonsupreme schools attached to duality, such as the school of the Vishnuite tantrikas—whom he describes as "practitioners of the path of the right hand."[50]

Lalla, the fourteenth-century master and poet, also recognized herself as a practitioner of the path of the left hand:

*Stand, Royal Woman,*
*Ready to offer wine, meat and pleasure!*
*If you know the supreme state*
*Everything is reunited in the heart of non-duality.*
*When you surrender to the celebration in the company of*
*    tantrikas*
*You glorify the Path of the Left Hand!*

Here is what Abhinavagupta writes:

The union with the yogini is of two kinds, according to whether it occurs by yogic necessity or by love. For the first, it is befitting to be attentive to her penetratable points, for the second, show creativity. . . . During union with the yoginis, one necessarily contacts consciousness, and for this reason this day will be considered a day of plenitude. One can say the same thing about the union between two members of the spiritual family.[51]

Later, Abhinavagupta clarifies:

Consciousness, which is composed of all things, enters into a state of contraction due to the differences generated by separate bodies, but it returns to a state of oneness, to a state of expansion, when all of its components are able to reflect back on each other. The totality of our own rays of consciousness are reflected back one on the other when, overflowing in the individual consciousness

125

of all present as if in so many mirrors, and without any effort whatsoever in an intense fashion, it becomes universal. For this reason, when a group of people gather together during the performance of a dance or of song, etc., there will be true enjoyment when they are concentrated and immersed in the spectacle all together and not one by one. Consciousness which is overflowing with bliss, even when considered individually, attains in these spectacles a state of unity and, because of that, a state of full and perfect blissfulness. The absence of causes of contraction such as jealousy, hate, etc., allows consciousness in such moments fully to expand without obstacles in a fullness of bliss, but if even one of those present is not concentrated and absorbed, then consciousness remains offended as at the touch of a surface full of depressions and protuberances because he stands out there as a heterogeneous element. This is the reason why during the rites of adoration of the circle (*cakra*) one must remain attentive and not allow anyone to enter whose consciousness is in a dispersed state and not concentrated and absorbed, because he will be a source of contraction. In the practice of the circle (*cakra*) one must adore all the bodies of those present because since they have all penetrated in the fullness of consciousness they are in reality as if they were our own body.[52]

In the introduction to chapter twenty-nine of the *Tantraloka*, devoted to the "sacred ritual," Abhinavagupta cautions practitioners who might not have the necessary qualities:

Now I describe the secret ritual according to the Kula method, which can only be practiced by masters and very highly advanced disciples. He who sees everything in this light and has destroyed all doubt is worthy of practicing this ritual. The Kula sacrifice can be performed in six different ways according to the circumstances: in outer reality, in energy, in a couple, in the body, in the vital breath, and in the mind.

For he who has not reached the heart of consciousness, the whole impulse of the senses, deprived of its sublime source, will lose all yogic efficiency: All the luminous rays of the senses, when they are deprived of contact with supreme consciousness, are immobile, stripped of their own nature and straining toward this supreme source.

Adepts, after having savored colors, flowers, and scents connected to the pleasures of dance and music, and after having consumed a light meal of food and drink forbidden by brahmanism—alcohol and meat—practice the yoga of lineage and pay homage "to the masters and to their Shaktis, who are overjoyed, without a defined body" and who are imagined in space. Next, the master draws a mandala, inside of which the deified participants take their places. Each area of the body is transmuted into a divine body through the means of sound (mantra) and through the touching of the various organs, head, throat, chest, navel, genitals, knees, and feet.

Then,

bursting with ambrosia and ardor, tasting their own juices brimming with savors, this appeasement finds its resting place by being poured into the Self. By the offering of their objects, the senses of touch, taste, smell, hearing, and sight become an overflowing stream that spills over, and by the fullness of the secondary wheels, and through the grace of a jolt of power, the Lord of the central wheel (consciousness) spills over impetuously.[53]

# 33

*A Tantric Path for the West?*

Our desire to reap the benefits of an ancient practice cannot be the object of a deal with the absolute. It is possible that we do not so much long to experience the ecstasy, peace, or joy of the mystics as, more simply, we desire to reach a state of plenitude and depth in our relationships with the world and people.

If we make this our objective, which is not divested of greatness, we are tantrikas in the making because we will discover that the distance between these two objectives is non-existent. As soon as presence to the world makes its home in us, we undergo a profound transformation that affects our whole being, body and mind. The breath will relax and find ease and plenitude; the body will let go, relax, and open itself to life; our senses will regain their marvelous functionings and serve as steedlike messengers to help us cross the dreary plains of absence. The motivation—as simple as it is essential—to escape from routine, from the cyclical aspect of our unhappiness and errors, which renew and prolong our suffering and our disillusioned attitude, is enough to send us gliding toward the experience of an immensely rich inner life.

The West is well armed for success. It knows well the devastation caused by everything about which the Orient can only dream. In a certain sense, we are lucky to have exhausted many of our dreams and to have returned, in a way, to square one. Because of this, we have the opportunity to procure for ourselves the most profound that life can offer us, on the condition that we break ourselves of our habits as consumers.

Tantrism is a marvelous approach to life, perfectly adapted to Westerners made weary by centuries of dogmatism, beliefs, and subjugations of all kinds. Our longing for freedom has been stripped of illusions. We are ready to stop trusting religious or sectarian institutions, which abound in the merciless struggle for power. We are ready to make ourselves heard on all playing fields in order to bring in the dawn of individual consciousness, which alone can eventually develop a collective consciousness. We have arrived at the individual maturity that can transform our quest into reality.

Finding a path stripped of all the marks of religious or sectarian fanaticism is possible. Allowing this path to be involved in each moment of our lives is also possible. All we need to do is reunite in one single body—ours—the divine, the temple, and the worshiper.

Through light and playful work, it is relatively easy to slip from general lack of consciousness to short stretches of presence, which little by little will give us the desire to continue in this direction.

When little islands of presence cut into our moments of absence, we start to taste the difference in pleasure that presence brings us. When practice mixes with pleasure, we are not far from being definitively lost to the cause of automatism.

Tantric practice is extremely creative. It is based, in the beginning, solely on the unhindered discovery of presence according to individual longing. As is written in stanza 74 of the *Vijnanabhairava Tantra:* "Wherever you find satisfaction, the very essence of bliss will be revealed to you if you remain in this place without mental wavering."[54] This linking of our everyday experiences within society to the divine, "the very essence of bliss," is one of Tantrism's great creations. No devaluing of everyday experience comes to set up a dichotomy between, on the one hand, the human being and his daily life and, on the other, his spiritual longings. Nothing is trivial anymore; everything rises to the sacred on the condition that our relaxed and easeful attention be such that there is no more mental wavering. This is the heart of the question. There cannot be both presence and cogitation.

Life is to be seized in its first moment of unfolding, in the luminous presence of *buddhi,* the intelligence that is beyond the hindrances of rumination, opposition, choice, differentiating judgment. If this tapping into reality brings us the serenity we are striving for, it is simply because mental silence opens to spontaneity, grace, fluidity, and joy. If the Tantric masters like to define themselves as *sahajīyas,* "spontaneous, awakened beings," it is that they have left behind all conceptual limitations of the pure and the impure, of the sacred and the profane. Everything is tremoring vibration and, in becoming sacredly tremoring beings, they open their heart to life.

This tremoring is accessible to us; it is not a yogic ideal. The *Spandakarika,* "the chant of tremoring sacred vibration," one of the most beautiful and most profound Shaivist texts, says: "Tremoring Sacred Vibration, the very site of creation and return, is devoid of all limitation because its nature is devoid of form."[55]

This absence of fixation is the very site of the spatiality that we can regain in a sudden impulse toward the depths of the Self. For this, let us jump with both feet into our daily life, let us allow consciousness to emerge naturally and re-place absence. These few seconds of consciousness that we will give to our life—thirty, fifty, a hundred times a day—are the door to bliss.

At the beginning of my practice with Devi, I had trouble thinking that things were how she presented them to me, close and absolute. I thought she was simplifying my work for me in order to lead me to a later stage of greater depth. This is the marvel of the Tantric practice, which right from the beginning recognizes in its practitioners their capacity to understand the most far-reaching of the teachings and which, in the presentation of these teachings, conceals nothing. Everything is told at the start. There is no progressive quest. The masters have always taken care that they could be understood by everyone, without book knowledge being a condition or requirement. These masters talk above all to the people around them, who are from all levels of society. They recognize no social, cultural, ethnic, or gender differences. Their teaching makes access to the philosophical texts optional. They are above all living examples of what they preach and happily, willingly, give the key to their realization: naked attention to reality.

What a practitioner of the Tantric path quickly feels, and sometimes the very first day, is that the benefit or reward—the state of joy, space, and freedom—is not subsequent to the practice of awareness. It is, on the contrary, an integral part of it. All I have to do is be present to any aspect of my inner life or to any event—it does not matter which—and I am right then and there in communication with what the teachings promise: openness, relaxation, ease, joy, love.

Everything is unceasingly within our reach. All we have to do is to reach out a hand and touch life profoundly. Each time this contact occurs, we come into a state of vibration and tremoring, we go beyond form, we penetrate to the heart of things, and we put our own heart into a state of vibration.

This continual vibration gives the extreme impression of being alive and in communication with all that is within our reach. The senses come out of their torpor; they stop waiting for exceptional circumstances to come along and wake them up. They find childhood again, adolescence, where the world unendingly sustains their capacity to vibrate. It is this deep and palpitating life that all those on the path of spontaneity know.

The main obstacle that the West will come up against is that what is presented as Tantra in our industrial societies is often an ersatz version in which all the basic principles have been twisted or distorted to fit with our most superficial longings for enjoyment, for orgasm. If we were to believe the newsmagazines, Tantra is "instant bliss"; a confused mix of 1960s therapies and spirituality with a light, Eastern scent. What we are fundamentally is not a perception, and it is therefore impossible to find through drugs, sexuality, or any sect or religion. It is not about undoing or disconnecting the intellect. Frustration affects only those who live in intention. This stimulation to try to do, to want to free the Self from thought and other childishness stems from a lack of orientation. In this approach we learn quickly to live in intimacy with the Self. This requires us to become familiar with respect. Just as you respect your environment in all its expressions, in this same way you respect your own limitations, the characteristics of your psyche, and those of your body. Here there are no fantasies of transformation, of becoming this or that, of arriving at such and such a psychic or physical result: You note things about how you function, about your intellect, about your affectivity. When you listen without intention, through pure love of listening, a clarity occurs, a space is created, you start to breathe. The rest follows organically. Respect, love of its expression: this is the Door.

Writes Éric Baret:

> As for finding an answer in Tantrism, we must not dream. The ritualistic practices, evoked by Kashmiri or other kinds of Tantrism, are reserved for those whose thought-sensory-processes are already highly purified. All caricatures of practices of this order, aiming basically for an exploration of sexuality, to reap further benefits from it, can only happen in a psychological, psychopathic setting. Sexuality and its emotional ramifications concern only the profane world.[56]

The advantage is that today—thanks to the work of such pioneers as Lilian Silburn, Ajit Mookerjee, Arthur Avalon, Swami Lakshmanjoo, Alain Daniélou, and Swami Muktananda, who have been taken up again by a new generation of seekers, some of whom are clearly informed practitioners such as Navjivan Rastogi, Mark Dyczkowski, Paul Eduardo Muller-Ortega, and Éric Baret—we have access to the authentic spirit of Tantra.

We can turn toward Tibetan Tantrism, Hindu Tantrism, Kashmiri Tantrism, Japanese Tantrism, Balinese Tantrism, or Chinese Tantrism. Tantric traditions such as those of the Naths are still very much alive today in Nepal, Assam, Bengal, and even the West. The Kashmiri masters who have fled their civil-war-troubled region have escaped to big cities like Delhi, Jamu, and Benares, or to Nepal. Some have remained in their hermitages in lost valleys.

The manner in which the Tantric masters teach is as original as their doctrine. They affirm that there is no fundamental difference between master and student, because consciousness is everywhere. It is enough to burn off the fog that keeps consciousness from manifesting itself. Their method of working is one long face-to-face: two individuals revealing themselves in total inner nakedness. Each master therefore can only teach a limited number of students so that this personal and individual contact can take place frequently. The greatest masters have hardly more than twenty or thirty serious disciples. They live with their family; a few students often stay with them or in the immediate vicinity. None of them has been tempted to develop a teaching that could directly reach hundreds or thousands of people, because the whole Tantric "flavor" would be lost in such an undertaking.

There is immense closeness between Tantric masters and their students. Interactions are devoid of anything ceremonial—which could bring to light illusory differences. The Tantric masters do not promote worship of personality. They have direct and simple relationships; they present themselves as they are, without giving rise to idealization. Love, no deference, no fixed attitude: This is what transforms aspirants of this most informal of paths. The student liberates herself by seeing herself just as she is—that is, naturally liberated, in the mirror that the master holds up to her. If we have the good fortune to be allergic to submission, to forms, to dogmas, to beliefs, to infallibility, to the idea of forming an artificial family isolated from society, and if we desire above all to live life deeply, perfectly integrated in society, then Tantra has something marvelous to offer to us. But Tantra requires a maturity, an independence, and a willingness not to conform. This is no doubt why so few people enter onto this path. As Lalla sings:

> *When differentiating mind is lulled and sleeps,*
> *The Kundalini awakens!*

*The five senses' source gushes forth forever.*
*The water of unceasing presence to the world*
*Is sweet, and I offer it to Shiva.*
*The unending sacred tremoring of consciousness*
*Is the supreme state.*[57]

# Part III

# 34

# Questions: Sexuality, Desire, Passions, Yoga, Ecstasy, Love, Joy, Pleasure, Space, Beauty, the Heart's Peace

*Why is there so much insistence on the body in Tantra?*

Without the body, there would be no philosophical or meta-physical questioning; there would be no creativity, no gods, no ecstasy, no yoga. The body gave birth to the absolute, and the tantrikas, by coming back to the embryo—the incomplete human form—regain the absolute in themselves in a constant outpouring of consciousness.

*What is the body?*

Space and all that it contains. The first thing a yogi experiences is that the body is not the image of the body. He becomes calm, he relaxes deeply, he starts to breathe, and suddenly all limits disappear. Each cell reintegrates space. This is what is called *samadhi*, experiencing union with the world. This experience can be very ephemeral, but it is what places the quest in its true location, space.

*I have followed all kinds of spiritual paths where women were allowed, but I have never felt that woman occupies a central or equal position. In other words, I have never had the impression that the divinity of woman was recognized. There is always subjugation to man. In the vows taken by the Buddhist nuns, for example, and in actual fact, a woman of a high level of realization always owes obedience to the less experienced monks. A nun is required to undertake a greater number of vows than do the monks, as if it were necessary to tame some kind of fatalistic nature. How has Tantrism been able to avoid this tendency?*

Shiva would be nothing without Shakti, the energy that puts him into the state of tremoring vibration. The worship of woman in Tantrism comes from the deepest and most ancient roots of this movement. Five, six, or seven thousand years ago, woman was worshiped in most cultures. The Great Goddess seemed to reign over the world. Even the Jews divided themselves into two opposing clans: those who believed in the Great Goddess and those who exalted a masculine God. There was a time when woman taught, carried the light. The Tantric movement has always worshiped woman because its most spontaneous and iconoclastic masters were often women, and the Buddhist tantrikas are no exception. The story is almost always the same: that of a great erudite like Saraha, Naropa, Luipa, Tilopa, or Marpa, who one day, after a dream or a vision, meets a woman, often an untouchable or casteless, who by the power of her presence and her state of realization, by her audacity and her humor, her disrespect and her incandescence, causes, in one instant, a scholarly and disciplined life to crumble.

All of these venerated masters recognized that the yoginis placed on their path were there to get them to cross over to the ultimate stage. When their universe collapsed they followed these women, leaving the luxury of the great monastic universities and the palaces where they were venerated in order to live lives of wandering, often in the cremation grounds. They received from the yoginis a teaching that integrated totality, and in turn became spontaneous beings. These extraordinary women, in Kashmiri Shaivism as well as in Buddhism, trained other women, and the lineages have survived to our day. There has never been a break in them. If we supposedly have more texts written by men, this is simply because the women most often sang spontaneous hymns and were not overly concerned about leaving a legacy other than the spontaneity that enables people to drink from the source. But this is in the process of changing, thanks to certain academics, like Miranda Shaw, who are doing marvelous work unearthing these chants, many of which have survived. The balance will be gradually reestablished. Still, what is important is that you, a woman of today, have access to this tradition; you can be one of these yoginis clothed in space.

*For a man, hearing all this talk about the supremacy of woman is a little frustrating. What about masculine energy in all of this?*

There is no masculine energy. There is only totality, space. The Tantric masters believe that a man who is alive, in a state of tremoring vibration, is a woman energetically. They believe equally that a woman who is not in this state of tremoring vibration is a man energetically. But this does not mean that there is any fundamental difference between man and woman; it simply means that everything is this tremoring vibration. The Tantras are written dialogues in which Shakti questions Shiva or the universe. At the beginning of most of the texts, it is stipulated that Shiva and Shakti form a single loving union and that they split apart from each other in order to give birth to the teachings. When that is done, they reunite. It is clearly specified that they are united "in the same knowing." In paintings Shiva-Shakti are generally represented as a single hermaphrodite body; when they are represented individually, there is always a sign of the other's presence, in the form of a serpent or the sun or the moon. Leave behind dual questioning; do not oppose the sun with the moon anymore: One could not exist without the other. Reintegrate totality at the body-mind level by abandoning yourself, surrendering, to reality.

*For several years I practiced another form of Tantra, which revolves much more around sexuality, and I must say that it helped me a lot. I had been totally absent from my body, and this training helped me get to know it. I think that one can reach ecstasy through sexuality without worrying about mystical or spiritual teachings, and that this is the fastest and simplest way in our current social framework. Why seek further?*

Who is seeking?

*I am, at least, I think . . .*

And what are you seeking?

*Ecstasy . . .*

What kind of ecstasy?

*The kind I experience at the moment of orgasm.*

Is that enough for you?

*I would like it to overflow a little, to become more long-lasting or permanent. Sometimes I dream of a kind of ecstasy that would influence my whole life.*

Then it is necessary to be involved in your whole life.

*What do you mean exactly? Could you be a little clearer, use regular words? I want to understand!*

I think you already understand, but let's look for clarity together . . . You say you have experienced ecstasy while making love . . .

*Yes, that has happened to me often.*

And you would like to experience ecstasy in other circumstances?

*That's exactly what it's all about, isn't it?*

Yes, that's what it's all about. When you have experienced these moments of ecstasy, how did they fade away?

*Soon after orgasm.*

So the orgasm was the ecstasy?

*Yes . . .*

And to have it again, what did you need?

*Other orgasms.*

Can you reach orgasm in another way besides during a sexual relation?

*Yes, by masturbation.*

What is masturbation?

*You know, you gently caress yourself . . .*

When you relax the whole body by the gentleness of the breath, when you abandon yourself, surrender, totally to gentleness, you will discover that the body is space and this is the most gentle of caresses, this is the most profound of orgasms because it gradually becomes established in continuity through the practice of presence to the world. Sexuality cannot be isolated, or made the special or choice vehicle of ecstasy, because the human being needs totality, he is totality. All searching that isolates one element of human nature in order to make it the only vehicle of the quest anticipates neurotic contact with life.

Sexuality is important if we believe that each and every contact of the senses with the world is a love affair. This is what the yoginis have taught us. This is what I understood from my time with Devi. For her, a leaf falling from a tree, a cloud passing, a fish in the river, the sensation of the sun or ash on her skin, the passing of an emotion or an idea—all that was lived like an unending love affair with the world. Every second, we are Shiva-Shakti in loving union; every second, our life provides us with a thousand propositions of ecstasy that a yogini does not let pass by because the flow of her consciousness continually inundates the tremoring, vibrating *yoni* of the world. To be this absolute lover in ordinary daily life is what causes wonderment to arise unceasingly. When the whole of life is permeated with this tremoring vibration, ecstasy is no longer linked to one particular activity: It flows in all things.

*I am homosexual and I would like to know if Tantrism has any position in regard to homosexuality.*

In Tantrism nothing is advised, nothing is forbidden, and there is no moral judgment—simply because we aim for full consciousness, and when there is full consciousness, everything is harmony.

In certain texts that concern the body and energy, it is said that sodomy is energetically disturbing, for both men and women. It is not said that this disturbance cannot be of use to yogis or yoginis. It is simply an observation. Dancing, breathing, looking, touching, listening also create an energetic and emotional modification. It is all about letting consciousness emerge in the body, in a more and more refined way, and about being in tune with the world according to one's desire, in freedom, creativity, love. Sometimes anal penetration brings peace; sometimes disturbance. It depends on the color of the sky, the hormonal cycle, the moon, that day's emotions, the season, the words, the vibration of the voice, the unconditional love that makes the body move and open or close its organs. All this is art; it is like the stream of colors that spreads out on the painter's canvas by the grace of a movement or an action freed of all intentionality.

*I would like you to speak about the satisfying of desire. Everywhere we look, it seems desire is the key element of language. Desire is everywhere: in ads, in magazines, in the way we dress, walk, laugh. We want to be desired, we want to seduce, at all levels. Everything seems like it's just a big game of mutual seduction, but sometimes I wonder if we can find satisfaction.*

Do you have the impression that you have found it?

*Yes, sometimes, temporarily, fleetingly, in simple things.*

Like what?

*This morning, I ate a pear that smelled delicious and was deliciously juicy and this brought me great satisfaction. I was totally happy and I think my desire was satisfied.*

You had a yoga experience. You fully connected with your desire; you let yourself be totally taken over by the qualities of this pear, and you found profound peace. But is it always like this?

*No . . . unfortunately . . . often, I don't find satisfaction. Yet I think I am passionate by nature and I search a lot, in everything.*

That's wonderful; yoginis and yogis are passionate beings. Why do you think you fail in your numerous attempts to have deep contact with the world?

*Maybe because of distraction, because of a kind of greedy appetite as well, like bulimia. It's awful—I want everything.*

That's marvelous!

*How do I keep this intense nature and find satisfaction? Are these things compatible or will the virtuous get the better of me?*

You have already escaped them.

*Huh?*

The true nature of desire is to disappear in the intensity of its search. If we offer it, as soon as the total freedom to act arises, we notice that it is self-sufficient, that it feeds itself on its own continual tremoring vibration because nothing else can satisfy it. Desire is a marvelous force that can flow from our heart in a continuous stream and shower over reality, ordinary daily life. To desire whatever happens: This is the playful, relaxed, easeful activity of the yoginis and the yogis, this is satisfaction in the continuous tremoring vibration of the human being, this is the joy of Soham, *I Am*. I am the source of desire, I am its path through space, I am its outcome, everything is alive, everything is only desire and satisfaction in one simultaneous tremoring vibration.

*Does the practice of nonpostural yoga that you teach affect physical and mental health?*

Every movement or action, every thought, every emotion,

every tapping into of our sensorality has an effect on our physical and mental health, because everything is connected. Even the way you open a door has a direct effect on your physical and mental health. When consciousness emerges, we encounter things with extreme subtlety and refinement of perception. The fact that Tantric yoga is the spherical unfolding of consciousness in inner and outer activity permanently changes our psychic and physical life.

*If this is the case, then the masters should never get sick.*

The masters are born and die. They get colds, break bones, have accidents, get seriously and not so seriously ill, they experience pain when they get cut or hit, but they do not turn the painful sensation into psychological pain. They live the pain in its real space-time, without prolonging it by mental activity. They learn to do this their whole lives. Life is extremely inventive; it always finds the means to prove to you that you are still a little rigid and tense, still projecting somewhat, still expecting a little, still somewhat vulnerable, and it is this constant dialogue with reality that keeps you from mistaking yourself for a master. Then, over time, it sometimes happens that certain people reach the absolute and continue to exist there.

*Do you mean that those who are considered masters do not have total mastery?*

They don't have it because they aren't looking for it. They accept reality, they go with life, they receive lessons from life and understand them often.

*Yet people rely on them!*

Rely totally on yourself, on your own capacity, on your own awakening, on your own consciousness, on your own sparkling jewel, and you will realize that you are no different from the masters whom you venerate.

*But you talk sometimes about impassioned worship?*

Impassioned worship is the creativity that allows you to discover your own completeness.

*Listening to you is irritating me to no end!*

Why?

*Because I have nothing the hell to do with becoming a yogini or a Siddha. There is already enough of this kind of confusion. You talk about things that are unattainable and for me, if I came here, it was to hear about things that are possible for ordinary mortals. I have a job that sucks, a pain-in-the-ass husband, a shitty apartment, a mother-in-law from hell, my car is a piece of shit that keeps breaking down, and I have friends who sap my morale. So make an effort: speak to an earthly woman!*

What do you like, what touches you in life?

*[silence]*

Really look . . . You wake up . . . what is your first calm or pleasant moment?

*I don't dare tell you!*

You mean when you go to the bathroom?

*Yes, I like it, I enjoy it.*

Me too.

*So we have at least one thing in common.*

Let's go on . . .

*After, I have to wait until my husband takes off. The morning is the worst. He doesn't say one word. He only talks at night. When he has left—I work later—I take a little time for myself. I really like taking my shower and especially washing my hair. I get the impression that I am washing away everything. That's one of the moments I like best. After, I put lotion on my body; that's nice too. Then I get dressed and leave for work. There I run into my boss and I shrivel up like an oyster.*

What do you think about when you wash your hair, when you put lotion on your body?

*I don't know . . . Sometimes ideas come to me, about work, or other things.*

And when you don't have these ideas, what happens?

*Nothing . . . I feel good . . .*

Do you think there is a connection between feeling good during these moments and your peace of mind?

*Yes, but I still can't find a cure for this sleepwalking.*

It's a cure for presence, a cure for consciousness, that Tantrism or Buddhism offers you. In these moments, you are totally present, you are a yogini.

*And what do I do to be a yogini when I am faced with my boss?*

How do you get to the office?

*I walk. It takes me twenty minutes.*

Is it pleasant?

*No.*

Why?

*Because I think about what's to come.*

Imagine for a moment that you are making this trip like every morning. What do you see?

*People who are aggressive and in a hurry, dogs shitting on the sidewalks, cars stuck in traffic, shop windows with things I can't buy myself.*

Is the sky still there?

*Obviously.*

Do you ever look at it?

*Yes. I see where you're going with this. Do I like it? Is it nice looking at the sky? Yes, okay. It's nice. And even clouds and even rain. I love when it rains on my face, people trying to get out of it and getting all stressed as if it were raining steel rods. I like the rain, especially in summer. And I also like trees, and every once in a while, I come across a little boy or girl who hasn't been gobbled up by life yet and I enjoy that, and every once in a while, I treat myself to a croissant and it's delicious and I pass by a florist's who puts flowers out on the sidewalk and I smell them and I even get a bouquet for myself every week, and every once in a while young guys try to flirt with me and that gives me a boost, as they say, and the first cigarette, that's good too, but it's not Tantric to smoke, they are only interested in nice things . . .*

There is nothing that is not Tantric.

*Even taking a drag off a smoke?*

If you are conscious of the pleasure it brings you, of the pleasure of each drag, it's yoga.

*So in the end, I might be a yogini?*

Each time that you are what you are doing, what you are feeling, what you are perceiving, you are a yogini.

*Even when I cry at the movies?*

Yes, because you have the courage to go with your emotions.

*What do I do about my boss?*

What don't you like about him?

*Everything.*

Can you find one good thing about him?

*No . . . I don't think so. . . . He's a sado-lewd-crude-yelling maniac and he smells like dirty socks. He has one thing going for him and that is that he leaves a lot to go have a drink, he's an alcoholic.*

When he's not there, are you happy?

*No, because I'm working.*

What do you do?

*Photocopies and parcels, I'm not very qualified.*

Have you ever let anyone else do the parcels?

*Yes, it's terrible, badly folded and badly tied. They don't stay together.*

So, you make nice parcels.

*Yes . . . I love the smells of the brown paper and the string. I think that, in the end, I really like making parcels. Are you going to tell me this is yoga?*

Yes . . . I think that you can find a deeper satisfaction in your work just as it is.

*Become a parcel-making artist, is that it? A paper and string yogini?*

The sky and trees, your boss not being there, a croissant, flowers, a break, a glass of water, a breeze, shampoo, body lotion, unhindered emotion, movies and cigarettes, defecation, and a look from a child or a man. If you do that, you have nothing to envy of the yoginis, and the more you do this, the more your realm of presence will grow, until the day comes when maybe certain aspects of your husband and your boss will touch you deeply, when your own openness will create theirs. But you can also decide to change jobs and to live differently. With openness arise movement and action, with movement and action arises life, with life arises the pleasure of presence to the world.

*So in the end, it's not so complicated.*

You have the openness necessary to live this experience deeply.

*I get the impression that in sexual relationships, and in life in general, we are a little lost because we no longer have ritual landmarks. We have abandoned everything, everything is a so-called open field, and in fact we are confused. What do you think about rituals—what is their function, and to what extent are rituals practiced in the path you teach?*

Rituals are in general codified rites of passage, of a basically magical significance. A ritual performed according to the rules, by someone who has the power to do so, opens new realms. At any rate, this is the way that ritual is viewed in most cultures. People consult oracles, they carefully choose a date, they prepare the instruments or tools, they purify themselves, and then they perform the magical act.

Tantrikas have a very different view. For us, there is no magic act because there is no duality and no intercessor. If we are what we want to attain, there is no need for an act that would open this unknown and far-off realm. No auspicious dates—all days are good from the point of view of consciousness—no instruments, no purification.

However, rituals do exist in Tantrism, but they are considered in a completely inner way. A ritual is not an action that will procure the divine for us, give us powers, etc. It is the celebration of the unity realized between the tantrika and the object of his awareness.

Ritual brings nothing: It is a celebration in honor of the state of unity in which the tantrika bathes. To take it farther, we can say that each gesture or act is a ritual celebrating union. Hence, there is no longer any separation between subject and object; everything is connection, everything is spherical, everything is plenitude.

In sexual relationships it is usual, for those who distinguish themselves from others under the pretext of following a spiritual path, to resort to a whole dramatic show: incense, candles, lights, music, joints, perfumes, soft cushions, shimmering colors, jewelry, and so on. This is fine—it can help people to relax, to come out of the mechanical aspect of sexual relations—but all this is like decoration.

What the other waits for is to be deeply touched in respect, tremoring vibration, spontaneity, nonprogrammation; with you, in contact with your body, she simply wants to get a taste of limitlessness. She desires you to be her and the creation of the sexual act to be a wonderment because it is always new, without reference, without past. Here is a very great ritual, that of a life, of a work of art. It can happen in a train, on a public bench, on the grass, or in a bed.

When you approach the other with this totality, you perform a very powerful ritual.

*I think I have sexual blocks. I went through psychotherapy, I consulted a sexologist, but my sexual life has not changed. I am extremely tense during sex, and it brings me absolutely no satisfaction. I think I have never had an orgasm. I was wondering if what you propose can eventually help me, even though I am aware that it is not therapy?*

Therapy is guided by specialists whose job this is, and it is centered on the idea that there is an *I*. The Tantric masters whom I have known are the opposite of specialists. They place everything in the perspective of consciousness and of the whole person in the abandonment of the *I*, which is dissolved by presence. One cannot replace the other, and to undertake a spiritual method in place of therapy is not a good idea. Sometimes our blocks necessitate the intervention of a specialist. This intervention allows us, when it succeeds, to approach *sadhana* more lightly, even more so given that this is a process during which our whole being will endure deep disturbances. On fragile ground, these disturbances can be devastating.

That being said, a sexual problem placed in the larger context is not a sexual problem; it is something that affects the whole inner dimension of the person and, even if this problem was caused by a very violent trauma—a rape, for example—it is possible that, placed in a larger, overall perspective, it would find the necessary opening and disappear. You have to really imagine that a person's quest, in a larger sense, gently reconnects the emotional and physical circuits that were left in abandonment or that never had the opportunity to become developed.

Female mammals spend considerable amounts of time licking their babies. The effect of this licking is to get the nerve endings functioning. No doubt, a very long time ago we also did this, since we rediscover this pleasure in sexual play. This is why the contact we all lack is so profoundly regenerating.

The fact that the Tantric approach does not include any taboos, that the body is viewed as something noble and pure, that disgust is one of the things we get rid of during *sadhana*, causes the body right from the start to feel accepted in its totality. Tantrikas specially honor the menstruating woman, because they believe her to be at the height of her femininity; she is seated to the right of the master in Tantric gatherings, and menstrual blood is a sign of unfolding power at its peak. Ascetics willingly use menstrual blood to draw on their foreheads the three symbols representing the Shaivist trident, the three energetic channels of the body, the three paths, and so on.

Woman is never impure; she is animated by a surplus of power. This shows an all-encompassing acceptance of the human being, of the body, of the sensations, of emotions and thoughts, of fluids, secretions, tissues, bodily matter, dreams, fears, inner space. This sole unconditional acceptance, which disregards the ordinary social criteria of selection, opens to those who feel themselves considered in this way an immense space where the body can find its own path of equilibrium.

This acceptance is enough sometimes to resolve serious problems; it restores to the person his cosmic facet. It can close deep wounds because being in *sadhana* allows the realization that at the heart of every person is an absolute and faultless realm that cannot be sullied or damaged by any action. All aggression takes place at the edges of this immaculate jewel. Sensing the existence of this jewel permits people who have suffered great violence, such as child prostitution, to regain, in the deepest part of themselves, a territory that has never been sullied. This provides an immense power, a freshness that nothing can ever touch, affect. Consciousness of this core is the most precious thing a person can discover, because he discovers it in himself, by himself.

When there is this recognition and this profound contact, everything can then regain the path of life and tremoring vibration. Contact with a master brings this certainty that we can find in ourselves what we were expecting to receive from a third party. This is extraordinarily profound, this sensation of total regained dignity, this sensation that emerging within us is the most secret place of our being, which is marked by nothing, which is love, spatiality, tremoring vibration. In the face of this shock, many wounds disappear. We come into contact, then, with a feeling of plenitude.

But there is a danger: that of attributing this rebirth to the master. That of believing that the master's actions have given us what we did not have already, which would put us in a place of dependence. As marvelous as your master may be, free yourself from the need to attribute powers to her. Everything breaks free from your own heart, no one gives you anything whatsoever, no one acts to provoke anything whatsoever. Love emerges from you because it is in you. A master is love, but she does not act: It is love that follows its own tremoring vibration, love that flows like a river. If, seated next to this river, you lean over its peaceful waves, you will see nothing but a stream of love—yours—which is reflected in the master's. At this point you will have discovered your own nature and your heart will be peaceful. You will have no debt toward anyone at all; only love spilling over in all directions.

*I hear you talking about love and it is refreshing, but what does one do when one lives alone? Can one find love without finding the other?*

That depends uniquely on the idea that you have of your body, of your limits, of the perception of your sensorality.

Are you the man whom we can look at, who can see himself in the mirror, or is your body something else? If you abandon tension, the image dissolves. If the image dissolves, your perception will fluctuate. Sometimes you will feel as vast as space, sometimes squeezed and tiny. You will develop a liking for the sensation of being vast because, in this expansion, you will lose your sense of ego and your sense of separation. When the sensation of being condensed and minuscule comes, you will be afraid you are going to disappear. But you will also find this fear reappearing at the edges of the feeling of expansion. Little by little, by playing with this fear, you will discover that there are no limits, neither in one sense nor in the other. Then, losing both the attachment to expansion and the fear of being infinitely condensed, you will start to perceive yourself as a mass free of all limitation and all fear, and you will be able to get a taste of a state of being in which solitude no longer exists because you will be totality.

*What way do I take to get there?*

You are the way and the destination.

*How do I start?*

By entering into profound communication with the reality of your life as it is.

*How do I find this capacity, develop it?*

By starting with what touches you or moves you naturally. If you are only that, even for a few seconds each day, your life will be transformed and the dynamic of presence will gain some ground with each new moment of full consciousness of this reality. Start each morning with the simplest things: a few swallows of tea or coffee, the taste of a piece of bread and butter, a few steps down the street. The pleasure of one peaceful breath. That is where we grasp the absolute.

*There exist other passions and other desires, like power and money. Can there be something positive in these forces that take us over, or do they have to be eradicated if we are thinking seriously about following a spiritual path?*

Nothing has to be eradicated. The classic trilogy—sex, power, money—requires a great deal of determination, a great deal of energy from its adepts. You have to be ready to suffer until the time comes when you have become desensitized. If this force becomes conscious of itself, of its real and deep desire, it will realize that these three passions are only masks, merely distorted translations of a deeper need, the need to be loved and recognized.

We imagine that we need to be loved and recognized as a totally unique being, as an entity separate from the common mortal by our greatness, and this also is a distorted translation of an essential need, the need to be recognized as non-separate from the world, as a stream of love independent of an elevated ego.

The ego is the part of the human body-mind most susceptible to elevation. We need to be recognized and loved far beyond the ego. This unconditional love alone liberates people. When this essential need is understood, power, sex, and money hold no more interest than masks abandoned at the end of a carnival.

The positive force of all the passions is that it can allow us to return to the essential source of the Self. Passions then become *the passion*. This passionate impulse can only be satisfied by the discovery of the incandescent core of the Self. This is the reason the Tantric masters have a predilection for passionate people, because only they have the force and the courage to go all the way to the source. All the great saints, in all the traditions, are beings who live absolute passion.

*Can you speak about the ideal relationship between master and student? What really happens and what makes this relationship different in Tantrism? Isn't there a risk of subjugation, of dependence?*

The ideal relationship between master and disciple is a passionate relationship that has regained the impulse of the original passion, that of the Self. It is a personal relationship, a long face-to-face, wherein each will totally reveal himself, without the least pretending. It is a stripping, cleansing relationship that breaks down spiritual fantasies one by one in a continual voyage toward the center where all differences are abolished.

Little by little the disciple recognizes her identity with the master and the universe; she ceases to be in a rectilinear dynamic and enters into a spherical effervescence where all movements or actions that are not circular, cyclical, will fade and then disappear. In a spherical perception of the world, all the concretizations that cling to the ego disappear, all differences fade, and the person reintegrates everything that has been extended without.

What is particular to Tantrism is the freedom of relationships. Nothing ceremonial, no fixed attitude: absolute love. We are not here to waste time with the expression of rigid forms. It is direct, simple, and without protocol. If fundamentally there is no difference, this must be apparent in actuality. A Tantric master is not afraid of showing his weaknesses, of being seen as he is. What he seeks to avoid is the dependence and subjection of his disciples, because in each particular relationship he fundamentally brings his own awakening to reality into play again. He shares fears, enthusiasms, idle times, boredom and discouragement, terror, in the very moment each happens, leaving the reassuring cocoon of the ego, the anxiety of abandon. He never acts the role of condescending guide; he lives what his disciple lives. It is the intensity of this relationship that causes the Tantric teaching to be given to only a small number of people. And in any case very few people truly want this intensity, because it leads to total inner nakedness. Most people are looking for something more bland and neutral, more comforting. In the end it can be said that the Tantric masters teach all those who have this absolute thirst. Very few people are capable of entering into a relationship of this kind once they really understand that no one will do anything for them, that dependence is a major obstacle to the relationship, that all the light will be found only within themselves. Most seekers do not have the maturity required to stop idealizing their master, to stop creating dependence, to accept their solitude. The jewel of the Self is found at the core of this solitude. This solitude alone connects with the world.

*Don't you find it pretentious to talk about disciples?*

Yes, I know, people prefer the word *student.* Yet it is the same word. *Disciplus* in Latin means "student." People admit that professors of caliber have disciples, that master musicians have disciples, that scientists have disciples, that great chefs have disciples. It is only a word. The Ch'an masters have a lovely phrase: They talk about *spiritual friends.* Let's be spiritual friends, if you prefer.

*Sensorality and sexuality are talked about a lot in Tantrism. Is this to say that the masters have sexual relationships with their disciples, as is often the case in other schools where sexuality is passed over in silence?*

The Tantric masters approach the human being in her totality.

They talk a lot about the senses, sexuality, and passion in effect because the puritan schools abstain from talking about these or talk about them negatively. This openness naturally leads to a very close, very intimate relationship between spiritual friends, where the body is reconnected to the fundamental tremoring vibration, but it is exactly thanks to the depth of this intimate relationship in perpetual movement that there are rarely sexual relationships between masters and disciples—outside the process of the initiation to the Great Union, which is given only in exceptional cases. Of course, in all the traditions there are always cases cited about "masters" who sleep with their students. We cannot carry any judgment. Sometimes there is abuse; sometimes a marvelous exchange. Sometimes it liberates, sometimes it blocks the movement of the quest. Acting the moralist serves nothing. Each case is unique. Among the Tantric masters I have always encountered an immense respect for the body, for the totality of the other—and a great subtlety and refinement as well. I have never seen a person used for personal ends, but I know this does happen.

Sometimes, chaste and virtuous masters who have scrupulously observed their vows for a whole life give themselves over to actions that are not necessarily liberating for those who endure them. But this mostly happens when there are frustrations brought about by strict vows. What would be serious in these cases is if we tried to justify the actions of the master—who in the eyes of some fanatical disciples would not know how to make a mistake, even if he abused the naïveté of some, even if he succumbed to pedophilia. Caught in this unhealthy dynamic, victims of sexual abuse seek in vain to understand what was the "master's" message.

Sometimes masters do in secret the opposite of what they teach. Sometimes those wrongly considered masters are nothing but egocentric manipulators. Sometimes, authentic

masters do things that seem condemnable but thereby transmit the most profound teaching. All these questions are en-
circled by a gigantic halo of hypocrisy. Sometimes masters,
in a nonsexual domain, require their disciples to undergo tests
that to us seem too violent but that get rid of the final blockages. Sometimes masters are possessed by "sacred insanity"
and liberate people through unbelievable audacities; sometimes they turn out to be the "regular" kind of insane, and
their actions are dangerous. May we each follow our own
intuition, without judging.

The physical closeness is a wonderful and divine game
that makes us discover space, but whose fragility is as great as
the possibilities. It is a subtle and complex relationship in
which mutual creativity is required so that the phantoms of
possession do not surge up. A Tantric master projects nothing, a disciple learns to stop projecting, and the physical intimacy is the marvelous and fragile ground on which this
apprenticeship takes place and where everything can happen
in grace.

It is an art, constant and absolute creativity, divine
tremoring vibration. This is the freedom that I lived with my
master, Devi. This is the freedom that I continue to live with
a few other people following this path.

*I would like to talk about a delicate problem that is at the heart of
conversations between women: We often share a certain sadness in
noticing that men do not bring us the enjoyment we long for. Of
course there are exceptions, but I think most women live in overall
sexual frustration; we end up becoming physically and spiritually
dried up and drained because we don't find the quality of connection that we desire, dream about, imagine. More and more women
are purely and simply refusing to have routine sexual relationships; it's like the rift is getting wider and wider. Where are the*

*men? Why don't they join us in this ocean of pleasure that we are capable of conceiving and sharing?*

Men are afraid. They are hiding. They are attached to values and attitudes that, for women, are peripheral. Men suffer; the superficial feeling of their superiority in all points of view is constantly undermined by a deep intuiting of the incredible capacities of women. They suspect that they no longer have a special place in the world. In close company with women, they are caught between an image of themselves that is crumbling and an anxiety about joining woman in her freedom, her courage, her worldly intelligence, her sensorality. Seducers lose the nerve to seduce; sexists lose the courage to affirm their views; men are expecting a sort of fantasized disaster, which woman would mastermind.

A tantrika worships woman because he recognizes her power. This recognition dissolves all obstacles, is the cornerstone of a deep relationship. As long as we have not recognized the power of woman, we cannot touch her and we cannot satisfy her. The great masters of the past who sought the teachings from the yoginis totally melted; they abandoned the whole reassuring and frozen universe of knowledge and authority because they recognized, right then and there, the power of woman, and they let themselves be led toward totality, the unsettling reunion of the body, mind, emotions, and space.

If we enter into the spherical universe, into the marvelous sinuousness of the total being of woman, we regain the suppleness of the newborn, joyous spontaneity, unprogrammed pleasure, slowness, the dawning of life in our organs, our skin, our gaze, our movements, our loving acts. At this moment man can again deeply touch woman; with her, he can become wave, curve, breeze, luminous spatiality. Woman asks for nothing else, and the man who touches a woman in this way satisfies her totally. It is a way of expression that, well beyond sexuality, touches the deep roots of the person. In this way man regains woman in himself, and the whole universe becomes Shakti.

*In Tantra we often hear talk about control of ejaculation, which would allow men to perform better as lovers. In your books, you also mention this technique. Is this really possible or is this yet another spiritual illusion?*

The words *control*, *technique*, and *performance* arise from a certain illusion, that of believing that a woman is longing for "a good lay." She is longing for much more than that; she is longing for a deep connection with the totality of her being. I understand that a person can be interested in the first point— I was interested in it myself—but some generous and tactful women helped me understand that this was a paltry performance compared to their deep longing. Sometimes, I understood it more directly. One day a woman literally knocked me senseless in the middle of one of these vain performances. I was very grateful to her for this.

If you are in this phase, which can open into something else and is not condemnable in itself, it is not necessary to turn to Tantra. American sexologists like Dr. Barbara Keesling have detailed some efficient techniques for control, which you can find out about in her book *How to Make Love All Night*, published by Grammercy in 1998. Know that you have to be ready to masturbate every day, her book in hand or on the desk, and to enlist the help of compassionate female helpers. It is work but, in practical terms, it is not ideal; what *is* ideal is the heart of the approach. Despite the highly practical side of this book, those who truly reach the goal are rare, quite simply because the goal is very partial and because it does not take into account the deep and larger longing of

woman. Holding back, performance, technique are profoundly contradictory to total pleasure.

If you are captivated by the Kashmiri Tantric teachings,
you will discover that the larger quest of the person leaves no
room for these slightly neurotic ideas. Apprenticeship exists;
it goes hand in hand with the development of a complete
yoga of presence, which it is impossible to attain as long as
you get fixed on objectives. Then, over the course of time,
you will discover total abandon to woman, which passes
through the volatization of fears, total relaxation, and absence
of plans. Then you will perhaps be lucky enough to meet the
man or woman who will open you to these sublime
abandonings.

*You often speak about creativity, art, aesthetic beauty, and grace in
human relationships. Is this a personal inclination or it is a kind of
Tantric predisposition?*

Both. The historical Tantric masters were artists. Not only is
music very important to them but so is poetry, aestheticism,
the formal beauty of creation, the inner tremoring vibration
caused by aesthetic emotion, the coming into vibration of
the person. There is always recognition in terms of beauty,
because beauty draws us into spatiality and dissolves the ties
to the ego. When we listen to music, when we are in front of
a painting, it dissolves us, and our sense of separation disappears. We are then in the tremoring vibration of consciousness; in reality, there is no more subject or object. Sensitivity
to art leads to acute perception of the beauty of everyday life.
At this moment our entire life becomes the expression of an
art that is perpetually renewing itself.

This love of beauty is what pushed the Tantric masters to
write their teaching themselves, in short texts, of great intensity, of a very rich power of suggestion. Presenting ideas and

philosophical concepts was not enough for them. They had a loving and sensual relationship with words, with language, with the profound dynamic between silence and space that underlies aesthetic form.

Once we penetrate deeply into the human fabric, comparisons with art become vital, because the tantrika's search is precisely to transform life into a work of art—that is to say, into the discovery of the profound relationship of individual humanity to spatiality.

# *Notes*

1. Stephen Larsen and Robin Larsen, *A Fire in the Mind: The Life of Joseph Campbell* (New York: Doubleday, 1991), 361.
2. *Dohakosa*, from "Saraha's Treasury of Songs," in *Buddhist Texts Through the Ages*, ed. Edward Conze, I. B. Horner, David Snellgrove, and Arthur Waley (New York: Harper and Row, 1964), 226, stanza 19.
3. Bill Porter, *La route céleste* (Paris: Librairie de Médicis, 1977). Translation from the Tantra/Ch'an Web site (Frequently Asked Questions).
4. *Buddhist Texts Through the Ages* 228, stanza 29.
5. Gregory Bateson and Mary Catherine Bateson, *Angels Fear: Toward an Epistemology of the Sacred* (New York: Macmillan, 1986), 64, 61.
6. *The Krama Tantrism of Kashmir*, vol. 1 (Delhi: Motilal Banarsidass, 1979), 4, note 2.
7. Ajit Mookerjee, *Kali: The Feminine Force* (Rochester, Vt.: Destiny Books, 1988).

8. See Daniel Odier, *Tantra yoga: le Tantra de la connaissance suprême* (Paris: Albin Michel, 1998).

9. See the translation of and commentary on this sutra by Thich Nhat Hanh, *Breathe! You Are Alive: Sutra on the Full Awareness of Breathing* (Delhi: Full Circle, 1997), 8.

10. Thomas Cleary, *Minding Mind: A Course in Basic Meditation* (Boston: Shambhala Publications, 1995), 92.

11. Sigmund Freud, *Civilization and Its Discontents*, trans. Joan Riviere (London: Hogarth Press and Institute of Psycho-Analysis, 1973), 1.

12. Abhinavagupta, *La lumière sur les Tantras*, chap. 1–5 of the *Tantraloka*, translated with commentary by Lilian Silburn and André Padoux (Paris: Institut de civilisation indienne, dif. de Boccard, 1998). English translation here by Clare Frock.

13. *Ibid.*

14. *Spandakarika, stances sur la vibration, de Vasugupta, et leurs glosses*, translated and with commentary by Lilian Silburn (Paris: Institut de civilisation indienne, dif. de Boccard, 1990). English translation here by Clare Frock.

15. See note 12.

16. Jaideva Sigh's translation is as follows: "When one experiences the expansion of joy and savor arising from the pleasure of eating and drinking, one should meditate on the perfect condition of this joy, then there will be supreme delight" (68).

17. See *Tantra yoga: le Tantra de la connaissance suprême*.

18. Jaideva Singh's translation is as follows: "'Knowledge, desire, etc. do not appear only within me, they appear everywhere in jars and other objects.' Contemplating thus, one becomes all pervasive" (94).

19. Master Hsuan Hua, *Sixth Patriarch's Sutra: Dharma Jewel Platform Sutra*, trans. the Buddhist Text Translation So-

ciety (San Francisco: Sino-American Buddhist Association, Buddhist Text Translation Society, 1977), 91–3.

20. G. W. Farrow and I. Menon, *The Concealed Essence of the Hevajra Tantra* (Delhi: Motilal Banarsidass, 1992), 165–6, stanzas 35–7. *The Hevajra Tantra* by D. L. Snellgrove (London: Oxford University Press, 1959) offers this translation (vol. 1, p. 92): "Without bodily form how should there be bliss? Of bliss one could not speak. The world is pervaded by bliss, which pervades and is itself pervaded. (35) Just as the perfume of a flower depends upon the flower, and without the flower becomes impossible, likewise without form and so on, bliss would not be perceived. (36) I am existence, I am not existence, I am the Enlightened One for I am enlightened concerning what things are. But me they do not know, those fools, afflicted by indolence" (37).

21. Swami Muktananda, *Nothing Exists That Is Not Siva: Commentaries on the Siva Sutra, Vijnanabhairava, Gurugita and Other Sacred Texts* (South Fallsburg, N.Y.: SYDA Foundation, 1997), 96.

22. *Minding Mind,* 42.

23. Jaideva Singh offers this translation (brackets are his notes): "Unswerving *buddhi* [i.e., the immediate and determinative aspect of consciousness] without any image or support [i.e., without an idol or *yantra* (diagram), etc.] constitutes meditation" (134–5).

24. Lilian Silburn, *Aux sources du Bouddhisme* (Paris: Fayard, 1997). English translation here by Clare Frock.

25. *Buddhist Texts Through the Ages* 227, stanza 21.

26. *Ibid.,* 238, stanza 104.

27. Jaideva Singh: "All contact with pleasure and pain is through the senses [and knowing this], one should detach oneself from the senses, and withdrawing within should abide in his essential self" (126).

28. Jaideva Singh's translation and notes are as follows (70–1):
    "Wherever the mind of the individual finds satisfaction
    [note 1] (without agitation), let it be concentrated on that.
    In every such case the true nature of the highest bliss will
    manifest itself." [note 2]
    Note 1: *Tusti*, lit. satisfaction, indicates deep, moving joy,
    not agitation of the mind. *Tusti* refers to that deep de-
    light in which (1) one forgets everything external, in which
    all thought-constructs *(vikalpas)* disappear, (2) and in
    which there is no agitation *(ksobha)* in the mind.
    Note 2: One has to plunge in the source of delight. One
    will then find that it is the Divine, the Essential Self of all.

29. *The Lankavatara Sutra: A Mahayana Text*, trans. Daisetz
    Teitaro Suzuki (London: Routledge and Kegan Paul,
    1973), 192–3.

30. *Ibid.*, 193.

31. *Les entretiens de Mazu*, introduction, translation, and notes
    by Catherine Despeux (Paris: Les Deux Océans, 1980).
    English translation here by Clare Frock.

32. Constantine Rhodes Bailly, *Shaiva Devotional Songs of
    Kashmir: A Translation and Study of Utpaladeva's
    Shivastotravali* (Albany: State University of New York
    Press, 1986), 50, 74–5. Daniel Odier used for the French
    of these poems *Les Hymnes de louange à Shiva*, trans. R. E.
    Bonnet (Paris: Adrien Maisonneuve, 1989).

33. Mahayanasutralamkara, XI 49, *Aux sources du Bouddhisme*.
    English translation here by Clare Frock. Dr. (Mrs.)
    Surekha Vijay Limaye in her translation of this text (Delhi:
    Sri Satguru Publications, 1992) translates this verse, seem-
    ingly incompletely and somewhat obscurely, as: "This
    mind develops itself accompanying the turbulence,
    enchained by the view of the self; one is impeded in ar-
    riving on that stage which is the order of the self" (196).

34. *Doctrine secrète de la Diesse Tripura*, translation, introduction, and notes by Michel Hulin (Paris: Fayard, 1979). English translation here by Clare Frock.

35. *Aux sources du Bouddhisme*. English translation here by Clare Frock.

36. *La lumière sur les Tantras*. English translation here by Clare Frock.

37. Miranda Shaw, *Passionate Enlightenment* (Princeton, N.J.: Princeton University Press, 1994), 88.

38. See *Minding Mind*.

39. *Passionate Enlightenment*, 92.

40. John Hughes, *Self-Realization in Kashmir Shivaism: The Oral Teachings of Swami Lakshmanjoo* (Albany: State University of New York Press, 1994), 40.

41. Kalou Rinpoche, *Luminous Mind: The Way of the Buddha* (Boston: Wisdom Publications, 1997), 236–7.

42. *Ibid.*, 233–4. Italics are Daniel Odier's.

43. *Lalla, chants mystiques du trantrisme cachemirien*, translation and commentary by Daniel Odier (Seoul: Points Sagesse, 2000). English translation here by Clare Frock.

44. *Minding Mind*, 86–7.

45. Translation by Mike Magee, from the Hindu Tantrik Homepage Web site.

46. *Paratrisika-Vivarana by Abhinavagupta: The Secret of Tantric Mysticism*, edited by Bettina Baumer, English translation with notes and running exposition by Jaideva Singh, Sanskrit corrected and notes on technical points and charts dictated by Swami Lakshmanjoo (Delhi: Motilal Banarsidass, 1988), 42–5. Footnotes within the passage are from this text, unless otherwise noted. Daniel Odier used *Abhinavagupta, L'essenza dei Tantra*, preface, translation, notes, and commentary by Raniero Gnoli; translated into the Italian by Mariangela Nughes Smidt.

47. *Vatulanatha Sutra*, translated and with commentary by Lilian Silburn (Paris: Institut de civilisation indienne, dif. de Boccard, 1995).

48. See the recounting of this initiation in Daniel Odier, *Tantric Quest: An Encounter with Absolute Love*, trans. Jody Gladding (Rochester, Vt.: Inner Traditions, 1997).

49. See Ajit Mookerjee, *Kundalini: The Arousal of Inner Energy* (Rochester, Vt.: Destiny Books, 1982); Gopi Krishna, *Kundalini: Evolutionary Energy in Man* (Boston: Shambhala Publications, 1997); Robert Svoboda, *Kundalini, Aghora II* (Paris: Le Relié, 1999); Lilian Silburn, *Kundalini: The Energy of the Depths*, trans. Jacques Gontier (Albany: State University of New York Press, 1988); Swami Muktananda, *Kundalini: The Secret of Life* (South Fallsburg, N.Y.: SYDA Foundation, 1994); Lee Sannella, *The Kundalini Experience: Psychosis or Transcendence?* (Lower Lake, Calif.: Integral Publishing, 1992); and Arthur Avalon, *Serpent Power* (New York: Dover Publications, 1974).

50. *Tantrasara d'Abhinavagupta*, translation and introduction by Raniero Gnoli.

51. Raniero Gnoli, *La luce delle sacre scritture*, *Tantraloka*. English translation here by Clare Frock.

52. *Tantraloka* 28:373–80. English translation here from Paul Eduardo Muller-Ortega, *The Triadic Heart of Siva* (Albany: State University of New York Press, 1989), 61–2.

53. *Tantraloka*. English translation here by Clare Frock.

54. From the Tantra/Ch'an Web site. Jaideva Singh's translation is as follows: "Wherever the mind of the individual finds satisfaction (without agitation), let it be concentrated on that. In every such case the true nature of the highest bliss will manifest itself" (70).

55. *Spandakarika, le chant du frémissement,* text Tantrique du neuvième siècle, de Kallata, translation and commentary by Daniel Odier (Paris: Le Relié, forthcoming).
56. Éric Baret, *Le sacre du dragon vert, pour la joie de ne rien être* (Paris: Voyageurs Immobiles, JC Lattes, 1999). English translation here by Clare Frock.
57. *Lalla, chants mystiques du tantrisme cachemirien.* English translation here by Clare Frock.

To learn about retreats and other activities
in the United States featuring Daniel Odier, go to:
www.danielodier.com

# Index

# BOOKS OF RELATED INTEREST

**Tantric Kali**
Secret Practices and Rituals
*by Daniel Odier*

**Tantric Quest**
An Encounter with Absolute Love
*by Daniel Odier*

**The Complete Illustrated Kama Sutra**
*Edited by Lance Dane*

**The Complete Kama Sutra**
The First Unabridged Modern Translation
of the Classic Indian Text
*by Alain Daniélou*

**Tantric Jesus**
The Erotic Heart of Early Christianity
*by James Hughes Reho, Ph.D.*
*Foreword by Matthew Fox*

**Tantric Orgasm for Women**
*by Diana Richardson*

**Tantric Sex for Men**
Making Love a Meditation
*by Diana Richardson and Michael Richardson*

**Yoni Massage**
Awakening Female Sexual Energy
*by Michaela Riedl*

**Lingam Massage**
Awakening Male Sexual Energy
*by Michaela Riedl and Jürgen Becker*

Inner Traditions • Bear & Company
P.O. Box 388
Rochester, VT 05767
1-800-246-8648
www.InnerTraditions.com

Or contact your local bookseller